Joint Commission
RESOURCES

Educating Your Staff

About JCAHO's New Accreditation Process

Improving Health Care Quality and Safety

JOINT COMMISSION RESOURCES MISSION

The mission of Joint Commission Resources is to continuously improve the safety and quality of care in the United States and in the international community through the provision of education and consultation services and international accreditation.

Joint Commission Resources educational programs and publications support, but are separate from, the accreditation activities of the Joint Commission. Attendees at Joint Commission Resources educational programs and purchasers of Joint Commission Resources publications receive no special consideration or treatment in, or confidential information about, the accreditation process.

Joint Commission Resources, Inc. (JCR), an affiliate of the Joint Commission on Accreditation of Healthcare Organizations (Joint Commission), has been designated by the Joint Commission to publish publications and multimedia products. JCR reproduces and distributes these materials under license from the Joint Commission.

Printed in the U.S.A. 5 4 3 2 1

ISBN: 0-86688-854-3
Library of Congress Control Number: 2003116967

For more information about Joint Commission Resources, please visit http://www.jcrinc.com.

TABLE OF CONTENTS

INTRODUCTION

A New Accreditation Process

Shared Visions–New Pathways®, the new accreditation process of the Joint Commission on Accreditation of Healthcare Organizations introduced in 2004, progressively sharpens the focus of the accreditation process on operational systems critical to the safety and quality of patient care. It represents a vision that JCAHO has with health care organizations—as well as with health care oversight bodies and the public—to bridge what has been called a gap or chasm between the current state of health care and the potential for safer, higher-quality care. The process also represents a new set of approaches or "pathways" through the accreditation process that will support fulfillment of the shared visions.

Continuum of Process Improvement

By now, your organization is probably familiar with the name of JCAHO's new accreditation process, Shared Visions–New Pathways. But there are still many questions about the reasons for such a radical revamping of the accreditation process and exactly how it will work.

Accreditation must evolve if it is to have continued relevance for health care organizations or credibility for the stakeholders—the public, health care organizations, government—who rely upon the process. The accreditation process established at JCAHO's 1951 debut served the needs of those times, as did the much different process of 1991. Now, in the twenty-first century, expectations have changed and so must JCAHO.

That means everything—including the format of the standards, the on-site survey process, and even the accreditation decision—is different. More important, Shared Visions–New Pathways is about shifting the conceptual framework from survey preparation to continuously improving systems critical to patient care.

To achieve this vision, JCAHO challenged old assumptions and substantially reengineered the previous accreditation model without lengthening the survey process. For example, rather than simply adding new standards or accreditation requirements to those already in existence, JCAHO looked at the process anew. Organizations now find fewer standards and more precise descriptions of compliance expectations. This reduction represents the efforts of JCAHO and an external task force to reduce redundancy and clarify existing standards.

JCAHO also moved toward focusing on patient safety and quality improvement. The Periodic Performance Review (PPR) uses technology to facilitate a more continuous, efficient accreditation process by incorporating an additional form of evaluation at the midpoint of the accreditation cycle. Your health care organization now has the tools to determine if JCAHO standards are being met 100% of the time and to develop action plans to correct any deficiencies. This process, conducted at the midpoint of the accreditation cycle, helps your organization know exactly where it stands and fosters continuous compliance with standards. While it does not lessen the rigor of the accreditation process, this powerful tool may lessen the need for consultants to help ensure consistent standards compliance within your organization.

Shared Visions–New Pathways

JCAHO created Shared Visions–New Pathways to support a better evaluation of safety and quality of care by achieving the following goals:

- Creating a more continuous process
- Focusing on direct individual care
- Focusing on issues most relevant to the specific organization
- Enhancing consistency in evaluation
- Encouraging organizational improvement rather than survey preparation

Shared Visions–New Pathways concentrates on following the experiences of individuals receiving care in a health care organization. By tracing the path of randomly selected care recipients from the time they seek treatment to discharge, surveyors will be able to examine how JCAHO standards are being put into place to produce good outcomes and reduce risks.

Surveyors use tracer methodology to validate the successful implementation of action plans and compliance with standards. For example, surveyors might select a patient admitted to the hospital emergency department with pain from a pressure ulcer. The surveyor would look at the patient's care in the emergency, radiology, and surgery departments, along with any nutritional/dietary consultation and specialized wound care services. The surveyor might focus on how each of these departments in the organization assessed the patient, eased pain, obtained a medical history, and planned for care. The surveyor also would return to the nursing unit where the patient resides to discuss the findings as they are exploring the care processes. It may be that a new theme or area of focus—such as infection control—emerges from this tracer process. The surveyor would then explore this new area more thoroughly and ask other surveyors at the organization to explore infection control in their tracers to determine if similar findings exist in other tracer patients.

Focus is on the actual delivery of care —not on design or potential. This focus, combined with presurvey data—such as performance measurement information, complaints, government sources, proficiency testing results (for laboratories), and accreditation history—feeds the Priority Focus Process (PFP) and helps guide the tracer selection.

In addition to tracer methodology, the other critical elements of the new accreditation process include the previously discussed major consolidation of existing JCAHO standards and introduction of a PPR process (for most, but not all programs), along with the use of data from multiple sources to guide the on-site accreditation survey. This process shifts the focus from a frenzy of survey "ramp-up" every accreditation cycle to continuous systems improvement by encouraging your organization to "live" the standards on a daily basis.

The on-site survey is focused on your organization's unique settings, services, and delivery of care, and surveyors evaluate actions taken to comply with the standards as part of the accreditation process's focus on patient safety and quality of care. The new survey process allows your organization to spend its time and money on improving the performance of the organization and not on the preparation of the survey. In today's health care environment, resources are scarce. Accredited organizations have made this clear, and JCAHO pledges to acknowledge this fact. This acknowledgement is the reason why the standards and accompanying actions are designed to serve as a management tool to provide guidance and direction to organizations in their efforts to provide safe, quality care.

JCAHO has devoted much effort to addressing all key areas where accredited organizations have identified opportunities for improvement. Active, ongoing communication with accredited health care organizations, state and national health care associations, the public, and other key stakeholders facilitated the redesign of the accreditation process under Shared Visions–New Pathways. JCAHO visited individual health care organizations, conducted market research, held town hall meetings, communicated frequently with key stakeholders and advisory and focus groups, and pilot tested the process. This feedback from thousands of individuals played a significant role in the development and testing of the Shared Visions–New Pathways accreditation process.

A JCAHO white paper was developed in 2000 and set out this vision for a possible future accreditation process. Fundamental to the future vision was enhancing the credibility and relevance of the accreditation process in changing times. In addition, emphasis was placed on creation of a model that is more data-driven, less predictable, and more customized to the individual organization. The 1999 vision also determined to address growing concerns by accredited organizations regarding the value of JCAHO accreditation as judged by a cost-benefit analysis. To that end, it was suggested that the redesigned accreditation process should accomplish the following:

- Increase the real and perceived value for accredited organizations
- Cause the public to have greater confidence that organizations are in compliance with standards at all times
- Be acceptable to deeming authorities and purchasers
- Decrease costs to accredited organizations
- Increase customer and staff satisfaction
- Support the perception among accredited organizations that accreditation is more of a service than a commodity

The original white paper proposed the development, testing, and evaluation of an operational model that would meet the goals set out by the vision and its guiding principles. Today that vision is being implemented with a redesigned accreditation process that offers enhancements in relevancy, consistency, focus, and meaningful education during the on-site process and the accreditation process as a whole. The launch of these innovations is viewed by JCAHO as a further milestone in the continuous improvement of the accreditation process. These efforts reflect an ongoing commitment to make accreditation more of a service than a commodity and to increase its value to all stakeholders.

Shared Visions–New Pathways shifts the view of accreditation as a snapshot that provides a somewhat narrow and time-limited understanding of how well an organization's systems work together to something more akin to a movie that provides panoramic insight into the organization's daily operations. This approach reduces the importance of scores and makes accreditation a true validation of the organization's continuous improvement efforts.

By emphasizing organizational efforts to deliver safe, high-quality care and by eliminating anything that doesn't contribute to this goal, health care organizations and other stakeholders can remain confident in JCAHO's "gold seal" of approval. These significant changes in the accreditation process promise to present both opportunities and challenges. Accredited health care organizations and stakeholders who rely on JCAHO accreditation can be confident, though, that the streamlined standards and survey process focus energies on what is most important—providing safe, quality care, treatment, and services to the American public.

About This Book

Educating Your Staff About JCAHO's New Accreditation Process is the handbook health care leaders can use to educate their staff about the new accreditation process, which focuses on providing safe, quality care as part of everyday operations. This book is designed to provide you with accurate and authoritative information about JCAHO's new accreditation process and how your organization is affected by and benefits from its implementation. The most important thing to remember when using this book is that staff do not need to be experts on JCAHO standards or accreditation processes. Staff should simply know their jobs and understand how they fit into your organization's efforts to deliver safe, high-quality care. This is the true focus of accreditation.

Chapters in this book are arranged by each component of the accreditation process. Each chapter explains the activity in full to give health care leaders a complete understanding of the activity and then identifies who in the organization will be the most closely involved in the activity. Chapters include ideas for disseminating information to staff members to help them feel more comfortable with the process, along with suggestions on getting staff up to speed without large time commitments, high costs, and confusion. Practical examples, including education strategies, samples, and illustrations, can be adapted to meet the unique education needs of your organization. Tip boxes for getting the staff involved complete each chapter.

Specifically, *Educating Your Staff About JCAHO's New Accreditation Process* explains the intent and effect of the following:

- A new accreditation process that focuses on issues critical to care recipients (Introduction)
- Assessing staff education needs (Chapter 1)
- The Periodic Performance Review (PPR) that supports organizations' continuous standards compliance (Chapter 2)
- The plan of action that is developed for each standard found not compliant in the PPR (Chapter 3)
- A Priority Focus Process (PFP) that integrates organization-specific data and recommends areas for the surveyor to focus on during the survey, giving organizations maximum benefit from the accreditation process (Chapter 4)
- A new on-site survey process that incorporates individual and system tracers, the use of ORYX® core measure data, and better engagement of physicians (Chapter 5)
- Evidence of Standards Compliance and measures of success (Chapter 6)
- Intracycle survey events, including random unannounced surveys, for-cause surveys, and extension surveys (Chapter 7)

Just as these elements of JCAHO's new accreditation process build on one another to form a complete process, the chapters in this book work together to provide a full picture. Each chapter is devoted to a specific accreditation pathway. Use *Educating Your Staff About JCAHO's New Accreditation Process* in conjunction with your accreditation manual, the Survey Activity Guide available on your extranet site, and the latest information published in *Joint Commission Perspectives®* to become familiar with and to stay up-to-date with the new accreditation process. More important, use this book to set the groundwork for continuous standards compliance and continuous performance improvement that increases the quality and safety of care, treatment, and services in your organization. Your organization can also use its accreditation manual to learn more about program-specific requirements. See the table below for a grid of program-specific requirements.

Program Applicability of New Process Components

	Components						
Programs	**Revised/ reformatted standards**	**PFP[1]**	**PPR[2]**	**ESC[3]**	**MOS[4]**	**Tracer Methodology**	**Decision Process/ Rules**
Ambulatory Care	X	X	X	X	X	X	X
Assisted Living				X	X	X	X
Behavioral Health Care	X	X	X	X	X	X	X
Critical Access Hospital				X	X	X	X
Health Care Network				X	X	X	X
Home Care	X	X	X	X	X	X	X
Hospital	X	X	X	X	X	X	X
Laboratory	X	X		X	X	X	X
Long Term Care	X	X	X	X	X	X	X
Office-Based Surgery				X	X	X	X
Preferred Provider Organization				X	X	X	X

[1] Priority Focus Process
[2] Periodic Performance Review
[3] Evidence of Standards Compliance
[4] Measure of Success

ACKNOWLEDGEMENTS

This publication would not have been possible without the assistance of many individuals who contributed significant time, energy, and ideas. We would like to thank all those involved in the development of the publication but give special thanks to Janet McIntyre for her excellent writing.

NOTE: Throughout this book, the terms *patient, individual,* and *care recipient* are used interchangeably to describe all recipients of care, treatment, and services in different health care settings. In addition, the term *care* is often used to indicate the entire spectrum of care, treatment, and services a health care organization provides.

CHAPTER ONE

ASSESSING STAFF EDUCATION NEEDS

As the new accreditation process is implemented, health care leaders are educating themselves on the new process and considering what information staff needs. A general knowledge of the new accreditation process is important because all staff members—from executives to front-line nurses to support personnel—play an important role in organizationwide efforts to deliver safe, high-quality care. JCAHO will evaluate these efforts through visits to care units, staff interactions, discussions with care recipients, and sessions with leadership and key functional staff.

The dramatic redesign and improvement of the standards and survey process sharpen the focus of accreditation on the care systems critical to the safety and quality of care. Now organizations will be expected to "live" the standards by integrating these important principles into daily operations. This means staff will need to accomplish the following:

- Show that safe, high-quality care is your organization's priority in all patient interactions
- Focus on using the standards as an operational guide, 365 days a year

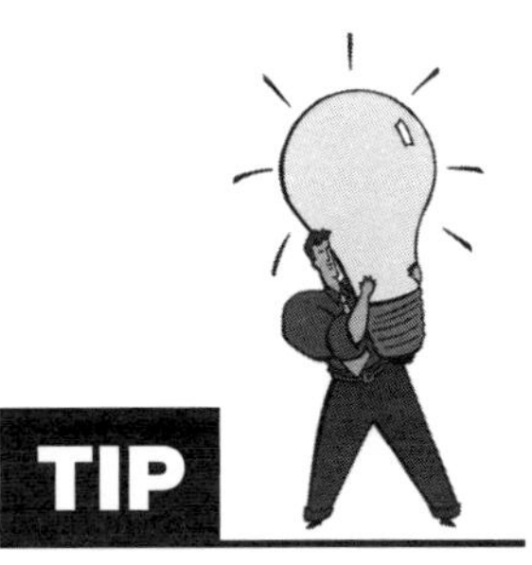

TIP

A special section on your organization's intranet could be used for educational activities. For example, previously asked questions could be posted with a simple search feature allowing staff to find answers to common accreditation-related questions. A list of resources, including Internet sites, educational organizations, health care associations, and electronic discussion groups, could also be included.

Staff Knowledge

Managing change is about managing expectations. In the case of Shared Visions–New Pathways®, the significant changes to the accreditation process promise to present both opportunities and challenges. Leaving behind the old and adopting the new demands the time, energy, and creativity of all involved. And it requires education about why this new vision for accreditation should be "shared" beyond both the boardrooms of JCAHO and your organization, to your front-line staff.

To effectively manage this process and reap the benefits for improved care, leadership must assess staff education needs related to providing safe, quality care as part of its everyday job. Staff will not be expected to know JCAHO standards or survey processes but they should understand how to effectively carry out their duties in a way that meets your organization's goals for consistently delivering high-quality care. Staff may want to know, "Will my daily work change as the result of the new JCAHO accreditation process?" and "Will Shared Visions–New Pathways change the way my organization operates?" The answer to both of these questions should be "no." JCAHO does not expect organizations or individual staff members to make significant changes as part of the new accreditation process. Instead, JCAHO has redesigned the focus of accreditation so that it reflects the way that organizations operate on a daily basis. This emphasis of the accreditation process requires no new preparation and is, in fact, dependent upon evaluating how your organization goes about providing safe, high-quality care in its everyday interactions with patients. See Sidebar 1-1 below for information on departmental information needs.

To aid in your communication with staff about the new accreditation process, see Table 1-1 for information that will help staff members understand their level of involvement in various JCAHO activities. You can customize the table to fit your needs. For example, create a department-specific table and only include elements that pertain to that department.

Sidebar 1-1: Do Certain Departments Need More Information Than Others?

It will be natural for some departments and staff at your organization to need more information about accreditation than others. For example, registered nurses may need more information than certified nursing assistants because of the former's supervisory roles.

To determine your organization's needs, consider the following questions:

- How does information about accreditation fit into daily operations and duties for both clinical and nonclinical staff?
- Are new staff members assessed for their need for information on accreditation?
- Do current staff receive ongoing information on accreditation as necessary to successfully carry out their responsibilities?
- Is information geared to specific disciplines or departments or units?
- How are materials or presentations tailored to specific disciplines or departments or units?
- Have staff been polled about what information they think would be most beneficial?
- Has your organization designated an individual as the in-house expert on accreditation?
- Has your organization designated experts in each department so that staff members can easily find answers to their questions and receive informal information as they carry out their duties?
- Do efforts to share information about accreditation as it relates to normal staff responsibilities include measurable goals?

Table 1-1: Addressing How Shared Visions–New Pathways Will Affect Staff

Components of Shared Visions–New Pathways	What It Is	Impact on You
Periodic Performance Review	A self-assessment of our compliance with JCAHO standards that we are required to conduct and complete between [*insert date*] and [*insert date*]	You may be involved in the Periodic Performance Review as part of your involvement in one of the following committees [*insert committee names*]. [*Insert name*] will lead the effort to complete our Periodic Performance Review. [He/she] will communicate to you additional details about this effort and how you will be involved.
Plan of Action	A brief and concise statement to JCAHO of how we will come into compliance with a standard	You may be involved in implementing the plan of action. [Insert name] will lead our efforts to carry out the plan of action and will be touch with all staff who will contribute to this effort.
On-Site Survey	Conducted by JCAHO surveyors, an evaluation of our direct care by tracing the paths of patients throughout our organization. The evaluation will be different from the old survey process in many respects.	JCAHO surveyors will spend much more time speaking with staff as part of efforts to look at how care is provided on a daily basis. You may be asked to talk about how you provided care for a particular patient. There are no "trick" questions, and you should not feel like you need to be a JCAHO accreditation expert. You only need to be able to explain how you did your job.

As another example, leadership at a hospital might explain to physicians that surveyors will want to talk with them during the tracer activity in the new accreditation process. Discussions with physicians about how their patients receive care will provide vital information to JCAHO surveyors as they look at how a hospital assesses patients, educates patients and families, respects patient rights, provides coordinated leadership, and promotes patient safety. Your organization's leaders can explain that JCAHO is reaching out to physicians to emphasize the vital position that physicians hold in a multidisciplinary health care team, providing clinical leadership and advocating safe, high-quality care for their patients. These interactions with JCAHO surveyors do not require special preparation or knowledge by physicians or staff; JCAHO standards should be carried out as part of regular work. The new on-site evaluation process, including tracing patients through their care experiences and talking with staff about those experiences, is the tool that JCAHO uses to evaluate compliance with standards.

Your organization can use this general idea to adapt messages for other staff in other types of settings, such as drivers at a home medical equipment organization, nurses at the ambulatory care clinic, therapists at behavioral health care organizations, and so on.

Frequently Asked Questions

After providing staff members with information about how their daily work meshes with the new accreditation process, the next logical step is to determine how staff members perceive the changes. Which areas of the new process are most important to them? Which areas present the greatest challenges? What refinements are necessary for reaching your organization's goals?

Handouts, an intranet section, brown-bag lunches, in-service sessions, videos, and other forms of communication can be useful in providing staff members with facts and dispelling any misconceptions that the new process involves new requirements or new ways for staff members to perform their jobs. It is also important to remember that there are no new requirements other than the PPR related to the new accreditation process. In addition, compiling a list of frequently asked questions, with honest, direct answers, can be useful in addressing staff concerns. For example, one of the most basic questions may be, "Are these changes really necessary at this time?" Explain clearly that leadership welcomes all questions and that team leaders are there to answer questions, too. Any questions that cannot be answered immediately can be documented, with responses to come as soon as possible. Two-way communication is essential during a time of change. By staying positive, focused, flexible, organized, and proactive, leadership can meet staff needs for information and foster an environment conducive to change.

In addition to answering specific questions, your organization may also want to reinforce earlier messages about accepting change. Staff needs to be reassured that it is natural to feel uncertain about change and that others across the organization are likely feeling the same way. In making a transition, your organization may want to encourage staff to let go of the past. This process could be something as simple, for example, as ceremonially tossing your organization's old JCAHO *Comprehensive Accreditation Manual* in the recycling bin and unveiling the new standards manual, or reminding staff that the main reason your organization has and continues to seek accreditation is to provide safe, high-quality care. Frontline staff members should be reassured that they do not need to do anything extra as part of the new accreditation process other know than know their own jobs. See Sidebar 1-2 for a list of values of Shared Visions–New Pathways.

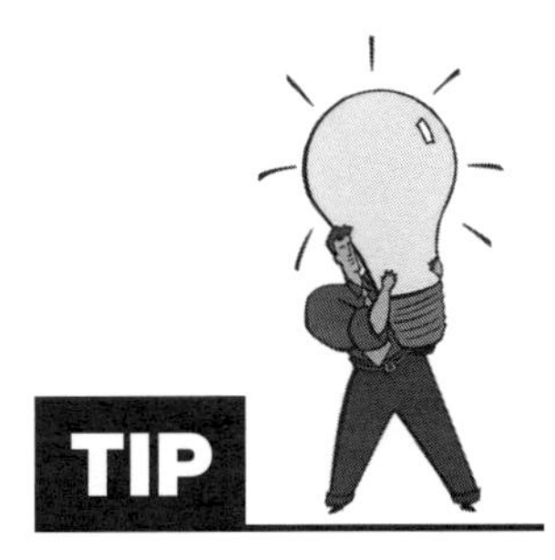

True learning will take more than one in-service training session. Consider methods that your organization can employ to teach a specific subject and reteach it in other ways. This approach will provide staff members opportunities to put what they have learned into action and then come back with questions. This approach also recognizes that education is a slow process that must build.

Sidebar 1-2: Value of Shared Visions–New Pathways to Accredited Organizations

- Greater relevancy
- Better focus
- Enhanced surveyor skill and consistency
- More physician engagement
- Enhanced customer service
- Minimize costs

Face-to-face interaction can help staff understand that the new accreditation process is unlikely to have any direct effect on their responsibilities. For example, a facilitator at larger organizations might lead focus groups, with representatives from each department participating. This type of gathering encourages staff members to be candid in their comments by offering a neutral moderator and the support of colleagues.

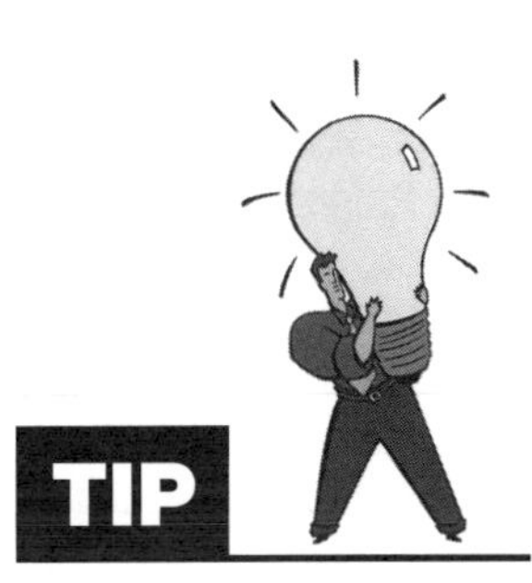

Encourage staff members to share their best practices with others in your organization. Staff tips could be posted on your organization's intranet, distributed at staff meetings, or included in in-service training sessions.

Common Misconceptions

One of the final steps in addressing staff information needs is to address common misconceptions about the Shared Visions–New Pathways initiative. While the name *Shared Visions–New Pathways* is likely familiar, there may still be many questions about the reasons for such a significant change in the accreditation process and exactly how it will work for your organization in its daily operations.

In addition to using information provided in this book and on the JCAHO Web site (see Sidebar 1-3 on page 15), it may be useful to explore with staff common misconceptions, including the following:

Myth: *JCAHO is attempting to engage in a game of "gotcha" with unannounced surveys.*
Fact: JCAHO is trying to shift the paradigm from survey preparation to systems improvement. The move to unannounced surveys is a logical evolution in the new accreditation process, which creates the expectation that organi-

zations will be in compliance with all JCAHO standards all of the time. By conducting surveys on an unannounced basis, JCAHO helps ensure that organizations that may be emphasizing major preparations for a survey only every accreditation cycle will shift to an every-day state of continuous compliance with standards.

Moving toward this goal will require your organization to work collaboratively across all departments and disciplines in order to be up-to-date on all standards, troubleshoot areas that present challenges, and resolve issues on an ongoing, timely basis.

During the on-site, unannounced evaluation, JCAHO surveyors will work with your organization to continually improve systems and operations, further eliminating the need for major presurvey preparations. Being ready for a survey at any time makes good business sense for your organization because it helps you to perform at peak levels and fosters safe, high-quality care. JCAHO also is confident that unannounced surveys will increase consumer confidence in the accreditation process and in accredited organizations, strengthening the value of accreditation for organizations. See Sidebar 1-4 on page 16 for information on unannounced surveys.

TIP

To familiarize staff with Shared Visions–New Pathways, consider the following:

- Regular e-mail messages from leaders
- Question-and-answer documents customized for your organization
- Articles in internal newsletters
- A Shared Visions–New Pathways informational booklet for distribution to all staff
- PowerPoint presentations
- Videos
- Informational letters to key constituencies, such as physicians or nurses
- Compliance checklists
- Games or quizzes that make the process a bit more lighthearted

Myth: *Unannounced triennial surveys are being conducted for all organizations, effective immediately.*
Fact: The new process will be phased in, with unannounced triennial surveys conducted on an optional, limited basis for two years. All such surveys will be voluntary until 2006. Up to 100 such surveys will be conducted in 2004, with the number of volunteer organizations selected increasing to between 150 and 200 in 2005.

Myth: *Random unannounced surveys will continue.*
Fact: JCAHO plans to continue to conduct one-day random unannounced surveys in a 5% sample of accredited health care organizations only through 2006, at which time all organizations should be cycled through the new unannounced triennial survey process. Organizations volunteering to undergo unannounced triennial surveys in 2004 and 2005 will not be in the 5% pool for random unannounced surveys.

Myth: *Shared Vision–New Pathways is going to mean more paperwork for staff.*
Fact: JCAHO is interested in how standards compliance benefits patients, residents, or clients. The focus of all accreditation efforts is on performance, not paperwork. The accreditation process will involve staff more directly by looking at how they carry out their normal work to benefit care recipients. See Sidebar 1-5 on page 18 for Shared Visions–New Pathways at-a-glance.

Myth: *The Periodic Performance Review (PPR) will reduce the rigor of the on-site survey.*
Fact: The PPR is just one component of a rigorous and fair accreditation

Sidebar 1-3: Getting Answers Straight from the Source

Frequently asked questions (FAQs) about Shared Visions–New Pathways are posted to the JCAHO Web site at http://www.jcaho.org/accredited+organizations/svnp/index.htm. These FAQs are updated frequently by JCAHO staff and provide a great resource for additional information about the Shared Visions–New Pathways initiative. If your organization has a question about Shared Visions–New Pathways, chances are that other organizations have had the same question. So visit the FAQs on the JCAHO Web site whenever you have a question. If your question is not answered there, you can submit your question to sharedvisions@jcaho.org.

Your account representative is also a great resource for any information you need as you move through the new accreditation process. As always, standards-specific questions should be directed to JCAHO's Standards Interpretation Group at 630/792-5900 or through its online question submission form at http://www.jcaho.org/Onlineform/OnLineForm.asp. FAQs about standards are also included on the JCAHO Web site.

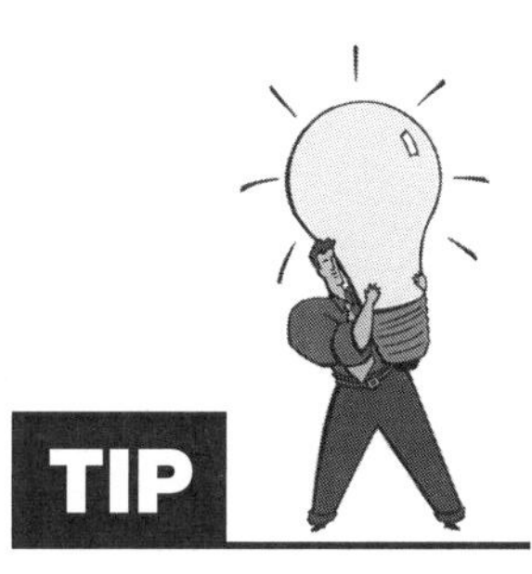

Consider asking all managers or department heads within your organization to focus on a particular topic during each staff meeting. For example, your organization's JCAHO coordinator or performance improvement team could create a list of relevant topics and a corresponding question-and-answer document or quiz for each subject. The information could then be used during staff meetings to provide an overview of the topic, explain your organization's approach, emphasize the importance to safe, high-quality care, and test staff knowledge.

process. The end result of the PPR—which can be thought of as an additional form of evaluation—will be a more continuous, efficient accreditation process. The PPR requires an honest, thorough evaluation that will challenge organizations, while possibly reducing costs previously associated with survey preparation. The new on-site survey process will continue to be a rigorous process that focuses on organization-specific, priority care processes and systems by incorporating information from the PFP to concentrate the survey on areas that are most critical to each health care organization's successful provision of safe, high-quality care. By adding a midcycle assessment of standards through the PPR, JCAHO moves health care organizations to a more continuous accreditation process—one that focuses on using the standards everyday, 365 days a year, as an operational guide to providing safe, high quality care.

Myth: *JCAHO wants to know only how we avoid health care errors.*
Fact: More than half of all JCAHO standards are concerned with safety because safety must be the first component of quality care. But it would be wrong to think that the only focus is on preventing errors; the standards and survey process are designed to help organizations do the right things right, thus improving the likelihood that care recipients will experience good outcomes.

Myth: *Without an accreditation score, we will not be able to measure or demonstrate success.*
Fact: Achieving accreditation is in itself a measure of success. JCAHO is eliminating scores in an effort to move organizations from thinking of accreditation as an exam with the focus on the best score possible. In addition, the publication of accreditation scores has led to confusion among both or-

ganizations and the public, who may try to over-interpret the minor differences—for example, between an organization scoring a 93 and an organization scoring a 95. The Performance Report generated in previous years has been replaced by the Quality Report. See Sidebar 1-6 on page 19 for information about the Quality Report. The true intent and value of accreditation are to continuously improve the quality and safety of care provided to individuals, not to receive a high score on an accreditation survey and then go back to business as usual.

Sidebar 1-4: Unannounced Surveys Set to Begin in 2006

In 2006, JCAHO plans to shift all accreditation surveys to an unannounced format. To phase in this process, JCAHO will begin conducting unannounced triennial surveys on an *optional* and limited basis in 2004 and 2005. Organizations wanting to participate will be drawn from a pool of volunteers that is due for survey in those years.

This initiative is designed to support the goal of shifting the accredited organization's focus from survey preparation to continuous operational improvement in support of safe, high-quality care. This change should essentially eliminate any perceived need for disruptive and expensive "ramp-up" for survey experienced in many health care organizations.

The shift to unannounced triennial surveys in all accreditation programs will be rolled out over 2004 and 2005, with full implementation expected in 2006. Implementation will be phased in to gain input from health care organizations participating in the early unannounced process, and to allow JCAHO time to develop the infrastructure to support these unannounced surveys.

The transition to unannounced triennial surveys in all accreditation programs for all resurveys is planned for 2006. All initial surveys will continue to be conducted on an announced basis to accommodate the needs of those organizations wishing to be surveyed as soon as possible after their request is processed.

To transition to unannounced triennial resurveys in all organizations, JCAHO will be required to make some changes to its infrastructure supporting the survey process. While the details of those changes will be worked out over the two-year phase-in process, some of the elements to be addressed include annual contacts between accredited organizations and JCAHO and timing of such activities as the Periodic Performance Review, delivery of priority focus tool output, and submission of demographic information about accredited organizations.

The Shared Visions—New Pathways model seeks to shift the paradigm of accreditation from a quest for scores through survey preparation every three years, to a quest for continually achieving and maintaining good operations for optimal care. The goal is to picture the survey as the validation of ongoing operational improvement, not as the lever for triennial change. Moving to unannounced surveys completes the paradigm shift and allows health care organizations to maximize the potential benefits of Shared Visions—New Pathways to their patients and, thus, to themselves.

Myth: *The ORYX® initiative to integrate core measures into the hospital accreditation process is being phased out.*
Fact: To improve the consistency of measurement collection requirements across accreditation and other oversight organizations, JCAHO has increased the ORYX® core measurement requirements for hospitals from two to three core measure sets. The sets—acute myocardial infarction, heart failure, community-acquired pneumonia, and pregnancy and related conditions—have not changed. Beginning July 1, 2004, surgical infection prevention will be added to this list. Data collection began with patients discharged as of January 1, 2004. This change is designed to minimize duplication of data collection efforts across hospitals and makes JCAHO measurement requirements consistent with those for the National Voluntary Hospital Reporting Initiative, a hospital voluntary reporting initiative led by the American Hospital Association, the Federation of American Hospitals, and the Association of American Medical Colleges and endorsed by the National Quality Forum. Hospitals will now be able to use measures from the same measure sets to satisfy JCAHO accreditation requirements and to participate fully in the National Voluntary Hospital Reporting Initiative.

In addition to addressing some of the common misconceptions listed above, leadership may also want to solicit unit managers and others for ideas about misconceptions specific to your particular organization. These false impressions can then be corrected.

Begin Developing Your Staff Education Plan

Your organization's JCAHO coordinator; patient, resident, or client services manager; and department managers—can help ensure success in your organization's accreditation process. Consider designating these in-house accreditation "experts," individually or as a team, to do the following:

- Develop and maintain a schedule of programs for staff members to attend on topics related to standards and performance improvement that will reinforce their efforts to provide safe, high-quality care to patients
- Assign a staff person to monitor the JCAHO Web site (http://www.jcaho.org) and to review issues of the official JCAHO newsletter, *Joint Commission Perspectives®*
- Register for JCAHO listserv announcements

Your organization may also already have an accreditation survey planning team. Be sure to ask these team members for advice on education and to solicit the active involvement of key stakeholders in the accreditation process such as physicians, nurses, pharmacy personnel, environmental services personnel, and other leaders who are in a position to facilitate and implement decisions. Also, consider including staff members qualified not by position but by expertise and experience.

Sidebar 1-5: Shared Visions–New Pathways at-a-Glance

- New standards format
- New scoring methods
- New survey techniques
- New postsurvey activities
- New accreditation categories
- New midcycle review
- New opportunities for the future

Finally, the following are some tips for success as you begin to develop your staff education plan:

- Consider educational programs that address evidence-based practice and clinical guidelines that support JCAHO's standards
- Consider collaborating with like organizations to share information through joint programs which might include a refresher course on the performance improvement plan, standards that are challenging for your organization or the field in general, new changes to the *Comprehensive Accreditation Manual,* and how the accreditation process will work
- Seek input from your line staff
- Identify systems introduced since your last survey, which may be affected by changes in requirements
- Focus on rationales and best practices for staff clarification and understanding
- Review *Joint Commission Perspectives®*, and the JCAHO Web site (http://www.jcaho.org), and Joint Commission Resources Web site (http://www.jcrinc.com) for current changes in standards that affect these areas and incorporate this information into your organization's staff orientation programs and competency assessments
- Possibilities for educational programs include seminars and conferences offered by the Joint Commission Resources Department of Education (http://www.jcrinc.com), state hospital associations, and professional associations
- Instruct staff about how to test all new policies and procedures against the standards and thereby identify gaps
- Offer opportunities for improvement, either in terms of quality of services or patient safety

Sidebar 1-6: Quality Reports Replace Performance Reports

One of the goals for the new accreditation process is to improve the value and relevance of the information provided to the public about health care organizations. By doing so, JCAHO hopes that it will help the public make informed decisions about their own health care. The main tool by which JCAHO will share this information is the Quality Report, which will replace the current Performance Report over the next three years. The report will be most useful in its electronic form, with links to definitions and additional information designed to aid in the viewer's understanding of the information. A print version of the report, as well as a users' guide, will also be available.

A Quality Report will be posted to an organization's homepage on "Jayco"™ 48 to 72 hours after an organization's full survey for only the organization to review. The report will be posted for public viewing on JCAHO's Quality Check® shortly after if the organization has no requirements for improvement. If it does, the Quality Report will not post for the public until after an organization's Evidence of Standards Compliance (ESC) is received and approved by JCAHO—approximately 90 days after an organization's survey is complete (45 days beginning July 1, 2005).

Because an organization must be in full compliance with all standards to achieve a decision of "Accredited" under the new accreditation process, there will be no scores for standards compliance in the Quality Report. The major sections of the report will include the following:

- **What is accreditation?** This section is a summary for the public on what it takes and what it means to be a JCAHO–accredited health care organization.

- **Summary of Quality Information.** This section provides an overview of all the quality-of-care components included in the rest of the report, including JCAHO-recognized quality awards, the organization's accreditation decision, accredited sites and services, and an overall assessment of an organization's performance against JCAHO's National Patient Safety Goals, JCAHO's National Quality Improvement Goals, and the Centers for Medicare & Medicaid Services' (CMS') Patient Experience of Care Results.

- **Detailed information.** Subsequent pages of the report give more detailed information about the organization's performance in different areas.

Learning the Language

Consider distributing a brief list of accreditation terms to staff to help everyone in your organization speak the same language. This list can be adapted to suit your organization's needs, and additional terms and definitions may be found in the Glossary of this book or in the current version of your accreditation manual. For example, a basic list might include the following entries:

Accreditation: Determination by JCAHO's accrediting body that an eligible health care organization complies with applicable JCAHO standards

Accreditation Cycle: A three-year period (two years for laboratories) of accreditation at the conclusion of which accreditation expires unless a full on-site survey is performed

Accreditation Process: A continuous process whereby health care organizations are required to demonstrate to JCAHO that they are providing safe, high-quality care, treatment, and services, as determined by compliance with JCAHO standards, National Patient Safety Goal requirements, and performance measurement requirements. Key components of this process are an on-site evaluation of an organization by JCAHO surveyors and a Periodic Performance Review (PPR)

Joint Commission on Accreditation of Healthcare Organizations (JCAHO): An independent, not-for-profit organization dedicated to improving the safety and quality of care in organized health care settings

Shared Visions–New Pathways: A JCAHO initiative to progressively sharpen the focus of the accreditation process on care systems critical to the safety and quality of patient care

Creative Team Activities for Problem Solving

Teamwork will be necessary as your organization and individual staff work to meet JCAHO standards in support of your efforts to provide safe, high-quality care. Teams can begin cost-effective performance improvement by engaging in creative activities such as brainstorming and multivoting to generate and narrow down lists of process-related issues, potential solutions, and approaches or options to address issues.

Brainstorming can be used any time a team needs multiple ideas or a fresh perspective. Brainstorming may, for example, be useful in using the PPR, an additional checkpoint in the accreditation process that helps staff to make sure your organization is on track with continuous standards compliance. Staff also may be directly involved in components of the new accreditation process such as the on-site survey, developing Evidence of Standards Compliance, and collecting data for measures of success.

To be successful in brainstorming sessions, all team members must participate, and a team leader should provide clear direction. Conducting an effective brainstorming session involves the following steps:

- **Define the Subject.** All ideas are valuable in a brainstorming session as long as they address the topic at hand. The group should be told that any idea is welcome, no matter how narrow or broad the scope, how serious, or how comical in nature.
- **Think About the Issue.** Allow enough time for team members to gather their thoughts, but not enough time to second-guess their ideas. Self-censorship can stifle honesty and creative thought.
- **Set a Time Limit.** There should be enough time for every team member to make a contribution, but not so much time that the team prematurely analyzes ideas.
- **Generate Ideas.** This part of brainstorming can follow a structured or unstructured format. In a structured format, group members take turns expressing their ideas in a predetermined order. This format encourages participation from every member but may result in a more pressured environment. In an unstructured format, group members voice ideas as they come to mind. This method is more relaxed but unless carefully facilitated it can lead to control by the more vocal members. No matter the format, it is crucial that neither the leader nor the other group members comment on any given idea. Reactions at this stage will inhibit and undermine the process. Be sure to write down every idea as it is stated. If a wordy idea is summarized, check with the person who offered the idea to make sure the summary reflects the person's intentions.
- **Clarify Ideas.** All ideas should be recorded accurately and understood by the group. There should be no attempt yet to rank or otherwise judge the ideas. Multivoting, which is described next, will help with that task.

Once the brainstorming session is over, teams sometimes are unable to quickly and easily narrow a broad list of ideas down to those that are most pertinent. Multivoting is a simple follow-up technique to review a long list of items and pare it down to a few manageable ideas that can be acted upon. After the brainstorming list is compiled, a designated team member guides the group through the following steps:

- Consider whether any items are the same or similar. Display the items under consideration on a flipchart. Eliminate duplicate items and acknowledge overlaps.
- Ask the team whether similar items may be grouped together. Faith in the process will be damaged if members feel their ideas are being altered without permission.
- If the group agrees, combine duplicate or similar items. All group mem-

bers—especially those who gave the ideas—should agree on the new wording.

- Number the items on the new list. Numbers will help the team readily refer to specific items on the list.
- Determine the number of votes each team member will have. One easy way to determine the number of votes each member will get is to divide the total number of items on the list by two.
- Allow time for group members to independently assign votes. Members are allowed to distribute their own votes any way they want. However, a team may decide that not all votes can be cast for a single item.
- Record each member's vote next to the items on the list
- Tally the vote
- Note the items with the greatest number of votes
- Choose the final group or multivote again. If a group of items is clearly the team's preference, this group is considered the final list. If votes are too evenly distributed, the team may multivote again, leaving out the two or three lowest items or reducing the number of points each member can assign.

CHAPTER TWO

PERIODIC PERFORMANCE REVIEW

JCAHO's new accreditation process is designed to help your organization maintain continuous compliance with the standards and to use them as a management tool for doing business and for improving care and safety on a daily basis. This process represents a paradigm shift for some organizations that may have "ramped up" operations a few months before their triennial survey, a costly process that can also put patient safety and quality of care in jeopardy. Organizations that focus on the standards only around the time of an on-site survey may miss important performance issues or opportunities for improvement that arise at other times. This process was put in place to improve the quality and safety of care provided by encouraging organizations to maintain continuous standards compliance at all times.

The Periodic Performance Review (PPR*) provides a framework for efficient and continuous standards compliance and focuses on the critical systems and processes that affect care and safety. PPR is designed to promote continuous compliance by assessing compliance with standards and Accreditation Participation Requirements (APRs) midway through the accreditation process. The PPR helps your organization to assess compliance, to develop plans of action, and to put those plans into motion. By participating in two thorough reviews of standards and systems throughout the accreditation cycle, your organization is more likely to incorporate the standards into routine operations.

Anytime individuals or organizations are asked to assess themselves, there is some question as to whether they will do a thorough and comprehensive job. Will organizations complete only a cursory review that indicates full or significant compliance with the standards and APRs instead of performing the suggested thorough review?

---

* The Periodic Performance Review is not yet required for all programs. Check your program's accreditation manual for your requirements.

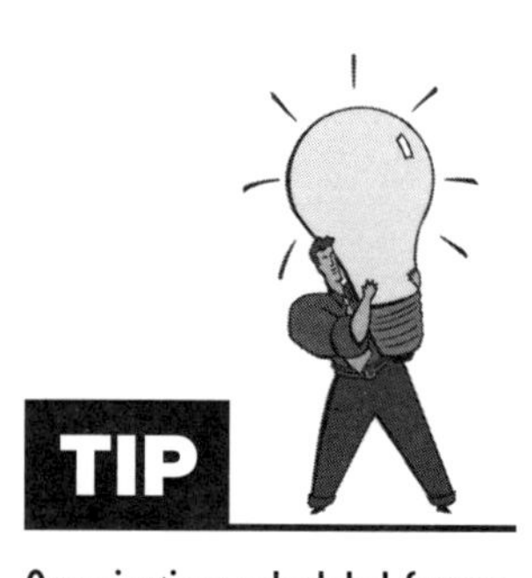

Organizations scheduled for survey before 2005 do not have to fulfill the PPR requirement. But you still might want to consider a self-assessment. Using the scoring guidelines within the 2004 accreditation manual, a standards review can be completed manually. Your organization can become familiar with the revised standards and assess your level of compliance. Also, look for a demonstration CD-ROM of one chapter in the PPR with the most recent version of your accreditation manual to get an idea of how the process works.

As you will see in this chapter, it is to your organization's benefit to involve staff in a thorough and honest assessment through the PPR process. Identifying problem areas, working with JCAHO on plans for improvement, and addressing issues in the 18 months before your next on-site survey make good sense for business and quality care reasons. The most significant benefit of doing so is that it fully supports continuous standards compliance and the improvement of safety and quality of care in your organization. Also, if your organization does not identify compliance issues in the PPR and these issues are discovered during the triennial on-site survey, your organization has only 90 days to correct the problem (beginning July 1, 2005, organizations will have 45 days to come into compliance). If your organization is not compliant with a standard, it will become evident during the on-site survey, and by that point you must correct the problem quickly or face a change to your accreditation decision.

An Overview of the Periodic Performance Review

The PPR is a new form of evaluation that is conducted by your organization and focuses on patient safety and quality-of-care issues. Your organization self-evaluates its compliance with all standards and elements of performance (EPs) that are applicable to the services provided and develops a plan of action for all areas of performance identified as needing improvement. JCAHO will work with your organization to refine this plan of action, discussed more fully in the next chapter of this book, to assure that its corrective efforts are on target. You will also be asked to identify measures of success (MOS) as needed for EPs with an MOS designation. This will validate resolution of the identified problem areas when the complete on-site survey is conducted 18 months later.

Your organization has choices about how it wants to experience the PPR. JCAHO will notify your organization via e-mail that it needs to identify—by the 15th month of its accreditation cycle—which PPR choice it wishes to use. The four choices are as follows:

- **The full PPR—**An organization conducts the PPR using JCAHO's automated tool, submits results to JCAHO via the extranet, and participates in a conference call with JCAHO staff to discuss plans of action and MOS for those standards with which the organization is not in compliance. The full PPR is the most common way to approach this process.
- **PPR option 1—**This option deviates from the full PPR only in the submission aspect. This option was developed due to concerns within the legal community and among risk managers in some accredited organizations about the potential discoverability of self-assessment information that is shared with JCAHO. While this option was created to respond to these concerns, most organizations have not expressed anxiety about the full PPR process and are encouraged to engage in the entire process. Under option 1, organizations must affirm that, for substantive reasons, they

have been advised by legal counsel not to participate in the full PPR. Organizations must affirm (using a screen in the PPR tool) that they have assessed their compliance with all relevant standards and APRs, developed plans of action for standards found not to be compliant, and identified MOS for all appropriate EPs. Organizations choosing this option will not be able to use the PPR extranet tool to score compliance with the standards. The scoring option will be disabled in order to prevent JCAHO from having access to the organization's scoring information. Organizations choosing this more limited PPR process will only be able to print the standards and EPs for the PPR from the extranet tool. During the next on-site survey, surveyors will request and review plans of action and MOS data to validate whether data indicate that performance has been sustained.

- **PPR option 2—**This option was developed to address concerns from some organizations that completion of a formal self-assessment of standards compliance, in and of itself, without submission of data to JCAHO, will still put them at risk for losing their protection from discoverability. Option 2 allows organizations to still benefit from a midcycle evaluation, and thus more continuous compliance with standards, without engaging in any activity that they think will put them at risk. An organization selecting option 2 when notified via e-mail of the need to make a choice will trigger JCAHO to schedule a survey at the midpoint of its accreditation cycle. All standards applicable to the organization will be subject to review, but the survey's scope will be limited and guided by the Priority Focus Process (PFP) output (see Chapter 4) and conducted primarily through the tracer methodology (see Chapter 5). The survey will be approximately one third the length of the organization's triennial survey. Organizations will be charged a fee for this survey.
- **PPR option 3—**If the organization selects option 3 as an alternative to the full Periodic Performance Review, it must attest that, after careful consideration with legal counsel, it has decided not to participate in the full Periodic Performance Review and instead intends to undergo a limited survey at the midpoint in its accreditation cycle. Following the survey, the organization may elect to participate in a conference call to discuss standards-related issues with Joint Commission staff. At the time of the organization's triennial survey, the surveyors will receive no information regarding the organization's survey findings under option 3.

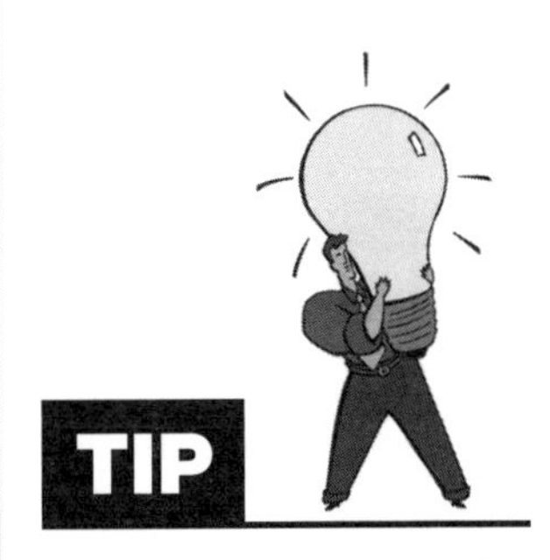

TIP

It will be important to plan ahead for the PPR. If you wait for access to the PPR extranet tool that becomes available 15 months from the time of the triennial on-site survey before you start planning, it may be too late to get the most out of the process. Careful planning will help you avoid feeling rushed and make the PPR process more meaningful to your organization. Reviewing the automated PPR tool in advance to become familiar with its features and requirements can be helpful in determining what PPR option to select, what approach to use, who will be involved, what data will be needed for the review, and what types of reports will be helpful.

If your organization is a hospital, you also must, in concert with the medical staffs, demonstrate that physicians were appropriately involved in the completion of the self-assessment component of the PPR (full and option 1) and in the development of plans of action for the full PPR and all options.

Note: The remainder of this chapter addresses the use of the full PPR and, in some cases, option 1. Please note, however, that even if your organization chooses options 2 or 3, for example, you can follow the tips outlined here to review your performance on a more consistent basis, not just before the triennial survey. If you choose options 2 or 3, it will be JCAHO that actually assesses you at the 18-month point.

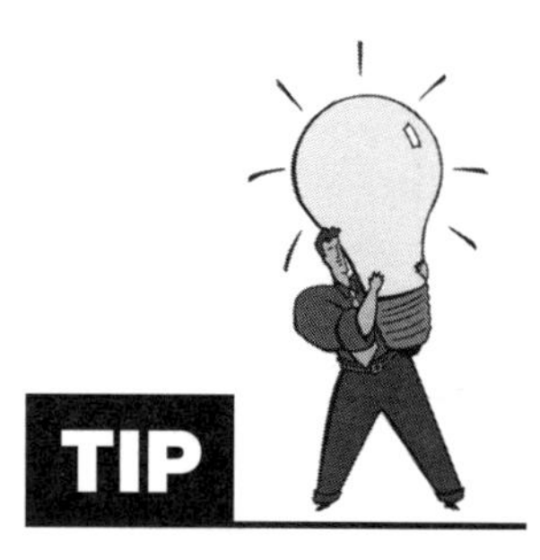

One individual may enter all of the information into the electronic PPR tool, or several people may be responsible for that job. JCAHO has no requirements on which method is used; your organization should choose the way that works best for you.

Completing the PPR

The PPR enhances the educational aspect of the accreditation process, providing an opportunity for staff to learn about strengths and weaknesses and to offer opportunities for improvement that are most relevant to your organization. The PPR tool will be customized to your organization, indicating which program standards are applicable to you, and will not allow you to submit your review until all standards are evaluated. The same rules surveyors use to determine standards compliance during your on-site survey are incorporated into the PPR. After you have scored all the EPs, the review tool will identify scored standards that require a plan of action. EPs that are scored as partially compliant but do not result in a standards-level decision of "not compliant" will be listed in a report for your reference. This report of supplemental findings will include standards where less than 35%, but some of the EPs for the standard are scored partially compliant, then they will be listed in an ancillary report.

It is important to remember that there are no penalties in the PPR for identifying areas of noncompliance. The ultimate goal is to help your organization achieve continuous standards compliance and to identify any areas that may hinder the provision of safe, high-quality care.

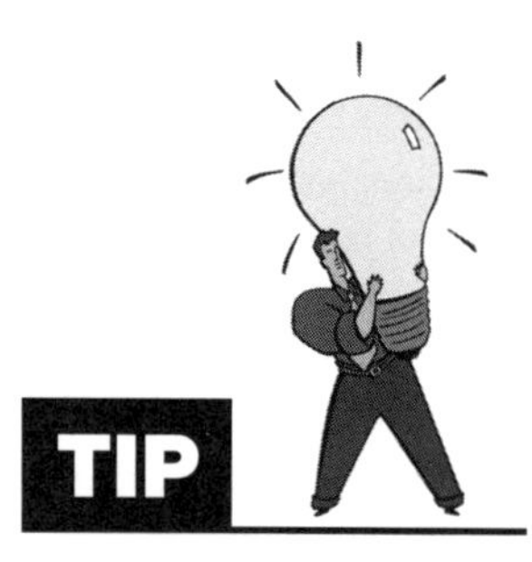

The PPR itself cannot affect your organization's accreditation status. However, leaders and staff should understand that failure to participate in the full PPR or in an approved option can affect your accreditation decision. When an accredited organization does not participate in the PPR, its decision is changed to Provisional Accreditation 31 days after the PPR due date. After 61 days, Provisional Accreditation becomes Conditional Accreditation, and after 91 days, JCAHO's Accreditation Committee will review the situation for possible Denial of Accreditation.

Once you have assessed your organization's compliance with all relevant standards and their EPs and formulated any necessary plans of action, you can submit your PPR electronically to JCAHO by the due date indicated. Within a few days of your submission, a scheduler from JCAHO's Standards Interpretation Group contacts your organization to notify you of a date and time for the follow-up telephone conference. Most telephone conferences will occur within 30 days following the PPR due date submission. Please choose two people from your organization to be spokespersons to the Standards Interpretation Group in order to facilitate the discussion. If you choose, you may switch staff depending on the topic being covered. However, no more than two people should actively participate in the call at one time. The only criterion for your representatives is that they should be knowledgeable about the information in your PPR. While only two people will actually take part in the call, you are encouraged to have all staff members listen in who are involved in the PPR.

Before the telephone conference, Standards Interpretation Group staff will review your PPR and any additional available background information to prepare for the call. You do not need to prepare anything for the review session, although your representatives should have a printout of your PPR with them during the session.

During the telephone conference, the Standards Interpretation Group staff member and your participants will go over each standard identified in your

PPR as not compliant, along with the plans of action and MOS you have created. The Standards Interpretation Group representative will either approve each plan or offer ideas about changes and additional suggestions. (Please see Chapter 3 for more information about the plan of action.) If Standards Interpretation Group staff members determine that your organization is actually compliant with a standard that you have marked as not compliant, the Standards Interpretation Group representative will update the PPR and note this in their section of the PPR tool that is returned to you. During the conference call, the Standards Interpretation Group staff member will also share information with your representatives on JCAHO's new scoring guidelines, helping them to learn what to expect.

After the telephone conference has been completed, the Standards Interpretation Group representative will post your PPR, including his or her suggestions and changes from the review session, on your organization's section of the extranet site.

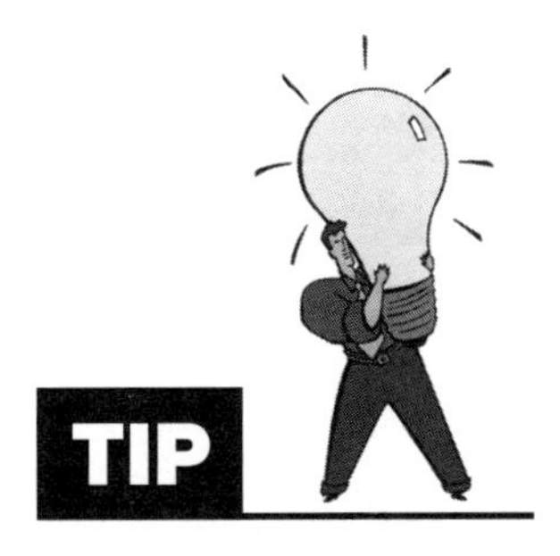

Expect the telephone conversation with JCAHO to go over the PPR to last between two and four hours. The length of the conversation with JCAHO staff will vary, depending on your organization's PPR findings and on the complexity of the plan of action. To ensure that ample time is available, schedule a four-hour block of time on the identified date. Also, please plan ahead because breaks will not be taken during the conference call, although participants from your organization may step out as long as it does not disrupt the conversation.

Educating Staff and Determining Staff Involved

To realize the full benefits of the PPR, your organization should take time before staff members begin the PPR process to help them understand how it works and how they will be involved. How prepared staff members are to conduct the review is ultimately more important than who is actually chosen to do the review. By knowing what to expect and what is expected of them, staff members can perform to the best of their ability. Specific topics to cover include the following:

- The goals of the PPR and how the PPR relates to accreditation and quality improvement
- How the PPR tool works
- What standards must be addressed
- What it means to comply with the standards
- How compliance should be assessed
- How to access information needed to evaluate compliance and to develop plans of action

The CEO or an individual designated by the CEO will submit the PPR to JCAHO, but the input of a variety of staff will be necessary to complete the process. Having your organization's staff conduct the PPR makes sense both financially and logically and provides many benefits, including the following:

- Flexibility in how the process is approached. The PPR is a dynamic process, and using internal staff allows your organization to customize the process as necessary.
- Enhanced individual learning by those involved in the process. By review-

ing and assessing all standards and APRs, your staff will become more familiar with them and what determines compliance. This learning process can result in continuous compliance and, thus, improved care.

- An opportunity for greater focus on areas of concern. Your staff members, more than anyone, are aware of problems and issues within your organization. This process gives your organization an opportunity to capitalize on staff knowledge in a positive, proactive way.
- An environment of open and honest discussion of concerns and problems can help reinforce a blame-free culture that is crucial in today's health care environment.
- Greater buy-in to improvement activities by staff involved in the PPR. By assessing yourself against all standards and EPs, staff will understand the need for improvement activities more fully.

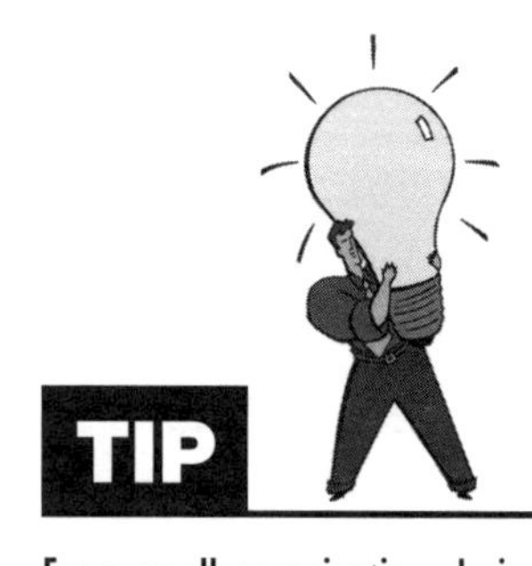

For a small organization, designating one individual as the project lead on the PPR process may make sense. This approach recognizes that staff is limited and the services provided are small in scope. Select a person with in-depth knowledge of the standards and their interrelationships. He or she will ultimately be responsible and accountable for the proper assessment of the standards and APRs.

Your organization may want to look at what it has done in terms of past self-assessments to determine which staff members will be involved in the PPR. Staff members responsible might include the JCAHO coordinator and members of the planning or performance improvement team. The PPR process also offers an opportunity to engage different staff in evaluating standards compliance. Involving supervisory staff and as many of your organization's clinical and other staff as is possible and practical is also a sound strategy. This process is a key way to educate your staff about standards requirements and how your organization is meeting them. It will also help them feel more confident during the actual on-site survey.

The PPR process is not designed to add more work to your organization's already full schedule. In fact, most organizations currently have some process in place to assess their compliance with JCAHO standards. The PPR just formalizes the assessment process and helps to encourage continuous systems improvement. That said, it will be important to schedule time for staff to complete PPR activities. As with any assessment process, staff may need at times to adjust schedules to have all key players involved. Staff completing the PPR will need to have time to examine intended practices or processes, to verify their implementation, and to consider whether your organization meets the EPs for each standard. In addition, staff must assess compliance with each APR, including progress toward the individual National Patient Safety Goals and their recommended actions. The results of this process will most likely be a list of areas that need improvement and must be assigned to appropriate staff members for improvement activities.

Depending on the size and culture of your organization, there are a number of ways to gather staff to evaluate standards compliance through the PPR. Some ideas include the following:

- Implement a group process that includes a multidisciplinary team or a department team that achieves consensus on compliance levels. For example, the health information management staff might assess the Management of Information standards, or the administrative staff might complete the Management of Human Resources standards. Or staff from infection control, medical staff, nursing, performance improvement, and environmental services might make up a multidisciplinary team that addresses compliance with a cross-department functional standards chapter such as "Surveillance, Prevention, and Control of Infection." Or an interdisciplinary team composed of staff members from different areas of your organization, such as registration, medical records, laboratory, surgery, radiology, and nursing, might review all standards and APRs, identify compliance issues, and develop plans of action where appropriate.

- Assign one or more staff to do a standards audit or a mock survey using a tracer patient. This staff person, for example, could be the JCAHO coordinator or performance improvement manager.
- Poll staff either through a questionnaire or in interviews and aggregate responses to identify standards compliance

All of these choices are viable, offering distinct advantages and disadvantages. For example, departmental teams provide varied input and offer greater review potential with a single focus. The disadvantages are that the review process might be inconsistent across teams within your organization, and there is a greater chance for redundant effort. The pluses of an interdepartmental team are a structured approach, shared responsibility, and multiple views of a focused area. On the down side, your organization will have to consider the time commitment, increased resources, and high need for coordination that can hamper interdepartmental efforts. Assigning a single person to conduct the PPR may ensure knowledge of standards, a simple reporting process, and defined responsibility and accountability but pose time commitment issues and create a single-dimensional review that leaves important constituencies out of this learning process.

Regardless of the staff approach taken, if physicians are part of your organization, then they should be a part of the PPR. To secure physician participation, your organization will need to show physicians how the PPR will ultimately affect and improve patient care. This approach can be accomplished through education at staff meetings or unit meetings. An interactive approach might be helpful, allowing for questions, explanations, and discussions.

By making an open-ended invitation to participate in the PPR process, your organization may not gain the physician support you seek. Expressing the benefits of participating in the PPR process, identifying the physician's role in the process, and estimating the expected time commitment of the process will help your organization gain additional physician support. Your hospital may wish to use physicians already involved with the process as champions to stimulate interest.

As with all staff at your organization, physicians have limited time for performance improvement. Organizations that involve physicians where their input can make the biggest impact on clinical care will reap the largest benefits of physician participation. Physicians on the whole are most interested in participating if they think they can make a difference in the health and safety of their patients.

Leaders also should play a prominent role in the PPR process. Leaders may include your CEO, administrator, governing body leader, senior managers, and any administrative or clinical leaders. These leaders will play a role in dealing with issues uncovered in the PPR, and plans of action may require ongoing leadership involvement and support. One way that leaders can get involved in the PPR process is to appoint an administrative sponsor or a steering committee that keeps other senior staff informed as to the status and results of the PPR.

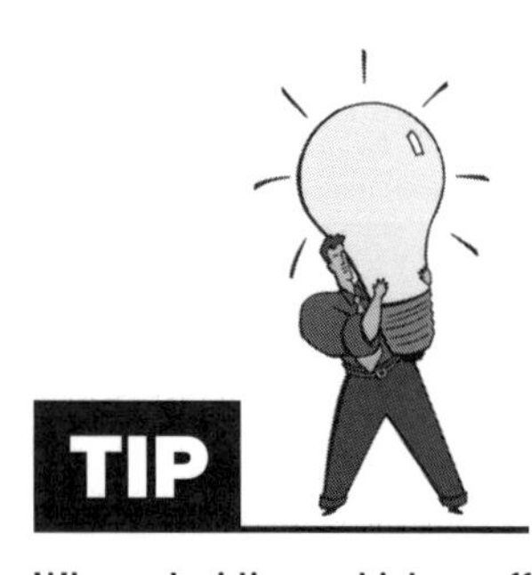

When deciding which staff should be involved in the PPR, remember that evaluating standards compliance is more than checking a box on a list or making sure there is a policy and procedure that covers the EP (although in some cases that is what a single EP requires). Staff reviewing compliance must be able to assess the process or system and the resulting outcomes associated with the standard. The real measure of compliance is implementation and outcomes.

Working with Staff to Develop a PPR Time Line

Your organization has three months to complete and submit the full PRR to JCAHO or attest that you have completed the PPR and that you have been advised by legal counsel not to participate in the full PPR and instead select option 1. This time frame offers a reasonable period in which staff can thoroughly assess compliance and develop necessary plans of action. Poor planning, though, can easily eat up this time.

In educating staff about planning for the PPR, set deadlines for completion of the components of the projects planned. For example, by the end of the first month, your organization may want to have the PPR team or individual lead selected. During that same period, for example, you may also want to educate all participating staff on the process and have an initial review of the first third of the standards completed. Or maybe your organization will decide to allow one month for planning, one month for the self-assessment, and one month for developing the plan(s) of action. Regardless of how your organization decides to divide the time, some thought should be given to how the three months will be spent. All staff members should be aware of the time line and work toward meeting deadlines. Leaders also must make sure that staff members working on the PPR are given enough time during their schedules to complete any work relating to the process.

Periodically throughout the PPR process, the PPR team or lead individual should report back to your organization's leaders to outline the status of the process and any issues uncovered. The frequency of these reports should be determined up front by your organization, and the PPR tool can help streamline this reporting process. Your organization may also want to distribute a formal, written report on the outcome of the PPR to leaders and staff. This report will help to emphasize the importance of continuous standards compliance and reinforce the idea that this is a team project. See Sidebar 2-1 for a staff primer on how to conduct the PPR.

The following is a time line for the PPR that may help staff to better understand this part of the accreditation process:

Step 1: JCAHO sends access information and instructions for the PPR tool to

Sidebar 2-1: A Staff Primer: How to Conduct the PPR

- Plan the assessment
- Generate a plan to evaluate your organization—this plan includes determining the approach; figuring who will conduct the PPR, along with how and when; reviewing the automated PPR tool; developing a data collection approach; and scheduling the assessment activities
- Conduct the assessment
- Report the findings

your organization at the 15-month point of your accreditation cycle, along with output related to critical focus areas and clinical/service groups (CSGs) from the PFP

Step 2: Your organization evaluates its level of compliance with all applicable EPs

Step 3: Your organization completes the PPR via the extranet. The electronic PPR will calculate compliance at the standards level based on the scores you assign to all applicable EPs.

Step 4: Your organization writes plans of action for the standards identified as "not compliant." You have three months to complete the PPR and develop plans of action and MOS, as applicable.

Step 5: Your organization submits via the extranet the completed PPR and plans of action to JCAHO by the 18th-month point of your accreditation cycle

Step 6: JCAHO staff schedules and conducts a phone interview with your organization if it has plans of action. At the point of PPR activity, your organization's accreditation status is not impacted by out-of-compliance standards

Step 7: During the full on-site survey, the surveyor validates the implementation of plans of action through a review of MOS information and an observation of the organization

Preparing for the PPR

In preparation for submitting the PPR, your organization may want to consider a review of how standards are being executed. Has your organization implemented processes to ensure delivery of safe, quality care consistent with the requirements of the standards?

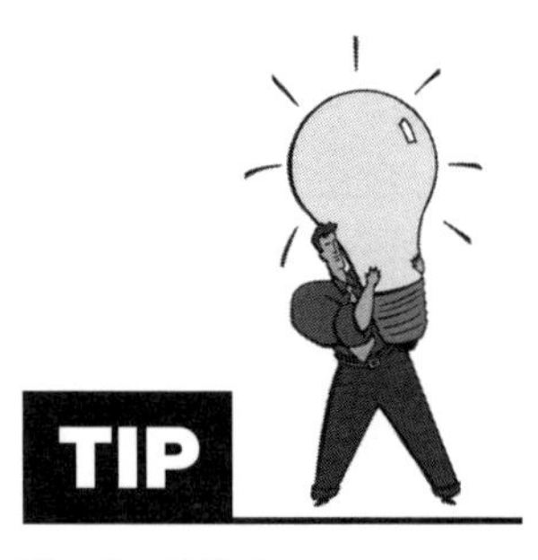

Tips for PPR Success

- Leaders play a prominent role
- Consider a steering committee to provide oversight
- Determine the best approach for your organization
- Establish the frequency of PPR reporting and meetings
- Educate your organization's internal "assessors" on standards and evaluation techniques

Staff members responsible for this task might include your organization's JCAHO coordinator, the CEO or administrator, managers, area supervisors, and performance improvement coordinator. When completing this process, consider the following:

- Make sure that a consistent process exists to review practices throughout the organization
- Review newer practices for topics or areas to identify other practices that may require changes in order to be in continuous compliance with the standards
- Be sure to review complaints against your organization, citations from federal and state governments, incident reports, and recommendations (both type I's and supplementals) from the last triennial survey
- If there are questions about standards requirements, JCAHO's Standards Interpretation Group is available for assistance through the JCAHO Web site. Select "Standards FAQs" and then go to the Standards Online Question Submission Form. You may also call 630/792-5900 and ask for a specialist.

Considering the types of data that will be needed to verify standards compliance may also give your organization an idea of staff members to include in the process. To prove standards compliance, your organization may have to gather evidence to answer a question, identify sample processes, or thoroughly review documents. The appropriate data will vary depending on your type of organization and the standard being examined. When possible, use existing data to help verify compliance. This approach will avoid extra work for your organization and provide insight into how staff are carrying out the standards to improve patient safety and quality of care on a daily basis. The following list provides suggestions on possible sources for such information and will help to determine exactly which staff are involved primarily or peripherally in the PPR process:

- **Medical or Clinical Records.** When such data are used, your organization should select an appropriate sample and establish reasonable thresholds for compliance. This plan offers many opportunities for caregivers—from nurses to therapists to home medical equipment drivers to dietitians to physicians to pharmacy—to be involved in the PPR process.
- **Policies and Procedures.** Again, simply verifying their existence and the content of the policies and procedures is not enough. The implementation is what is most important. This effort can include staff or managers from virtually every department—housekeeping, radiology, administration, and so forth—in your organization.
- **Human Resources Data.** These data may include personnel files, performance reviews, and orientation surveys. This plan presents an opportunity for the director of human resources to be involved in the PPR.

- Meeting minutes
- Interviews with key staff, management, leadership
- Surveys of staff, patients, and the community
- Building tours
- Drills
- Planning documents
- Performance improvement data
- Infection control data
- **Statement of Conditions™ (SOC).** This statement can help verify compliance with Environment of Care standards and identify any violations of the *Life Safety Code®*.*
- **The Medical Record Delinquency Form** (a blank form is available at http://www.jcaho.org).
- **Mock Surveys.** Although a mock survey may result in slightly more work for your organization, it will provide a true picture of standards compliance and highlight any issues that need to be addressed. As part of this mock survey process, your organization may choose to select mock tracers—those individuals who represent a CSG for your facility—and "trace" them through the care process. (For more information on CSGs, *see* Chapter 4. For more information on the tracer process, *see* Chapter 5.)

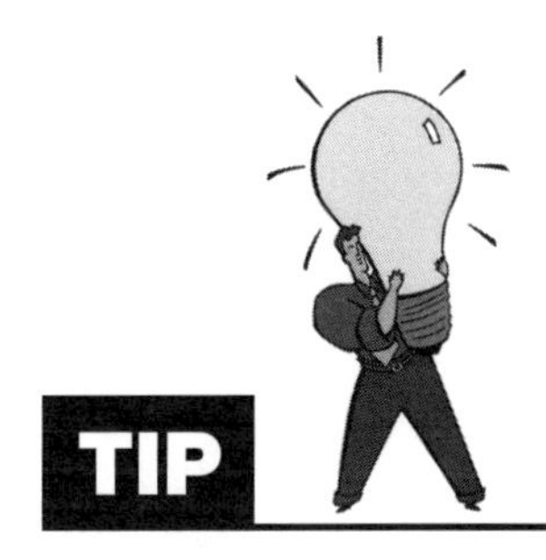

The "Messages" section of the PPR tool provides your organization with an area in which to check messages from JCAHO. Messages might include a reminder of your organization's PPR due date, the time remaining until the due date, or the status of your PPR once it has been submitted.

Getting Help

JCAHO offers a number of tools to help your organization assess standards compliance during the PPR process. For example, under the "References" section in the electronic PPR tool, you can click on the "Rationale" button to see information that helps clarify the meaning of the standard. You can also find a scoring guide within the "References" section that will help you determine what quantitative measures constitute compliance. Finally, you can click the "User Manual" tab in the PPR extranet tool for assistance.

* *Life Safety Code®* is a registered trademark of the National Fire Protection Association, Quincy, Massachusetts.

CHAPTER THREE

PLAN OF ACTION

After assessing standards compliance through the Periodic Performance Review (PPR) at the midpoint of the accreditation cycle, your organization is now ready to develop any necessary plans of action. Every standard that is identified as out of compliance requires that you look at elements of performance (EPs) and determine the problem, the solution, and the time frame for implementing corrective actions and measuring improvement through any required measures of success (MOS). In other words, your organization will need to develop a brief and concise statement to JCAHO that explains how you will come into compliance with a particular standard. This information will be sent to JCAHO electronically with the PPR, giving the Standards Interpretation Group (SIG) representative the basis for a follow-up telephone discussion.

Your organization can decide how best to go about the process of developing plans of action. For example, you may decide to complete each required plan of action as you work, standard by standard, through the PPR process, or you may opt to write all plans of action after all standards have been assessed. Either way, the idea is to correct any areas identified as out of compliance. See Sidebar 3-1 on page 36 for sample strategies for the plan of action.

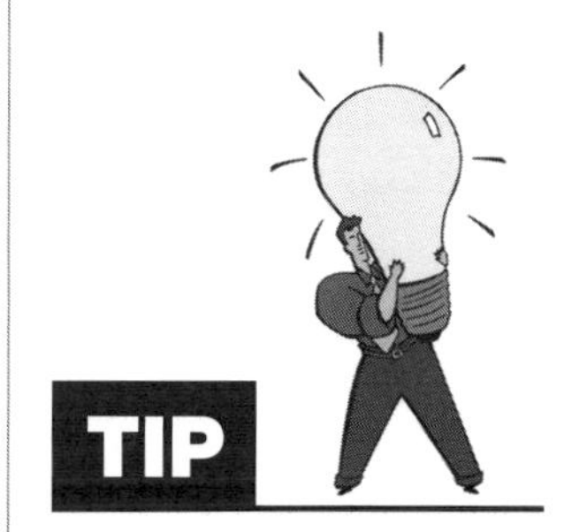

The plan of action process offers a number of benefits to your organization. First, it provides an opportunity to talk with JCAHO staff to determine whether your organization's strategy will help you meet the requirements of the standards. Creating and implementing the plan of action also encourages staff participation in and ownership of quality and safety activities.

Developing a Plan of Action

To ensure that plans of action are to-the-point, the PPR tool allows limited space for documenting your strategy. Your organization will have to be succinct in its descriptions while providing some detail and a thorough outline. For example, you may not be able to include large amounts of data and information in the plan, but simply stating that a policy or procedure will be created to address noncompliance is typically not sufficient.

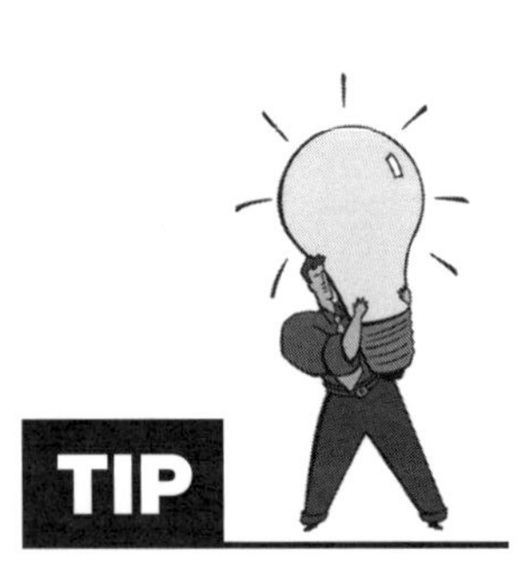

Hold brainstorming sessions to create your organization's plan of action. Gather staff from relevant departments and use a flipchart to write out the issue (standards compliance) in a simple sentence or two. Then ask who should be involved in developing and implementing the plan of action. Also, ask how your organization will measure progress in implementing each plan.

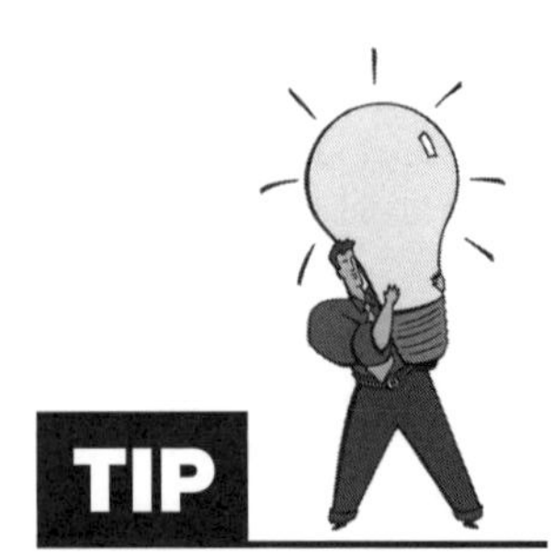

Staff completing the plan of action should include the facts and consider the who, what, when, and how.

Sidebar 3-1: Sample Strategy for the Plan of Action

- Designate one or two key people in your organization to oversee the plan of action process to eliminate confusion and duplication of work
- Designate staff members who are responsible for integrating information from multiple sites or services if yours is a complex organization
- Create phone/e-mail lists of key staff members involved in the plan of action
- Plan biweekly meetings involving key staff. These meetings can be in person or by conference call if necessary for your organization.
- Distribute minutes from these meetings to all staff members involved in the plan of action
- Start the planning process
- Allow time for all PPR leaders to review your plans and results before sending the plan of action to JCAHO

Your organization may want to create a written plan that is detailed yet brief, or you may wish to simplify the plan even further by using bullet points and shorter phrases. To create a successful plan of action, your organization should consider the following elements:

- The PPR tool accepts alpha and numeric characters so that your organization can identify the people responsible for carrying out the plan code or number. For example, your organization may discover noncompliance with a Provision of Care, Treatment, and Services standard requiring initial assessments to be performed as defined by your organization. To ensure that each individual's initial assessment is conducted within the time frame specified by the care recipient's needs, your organization's policy, and law and regulation, you may enter, for example, "director of nursing" as the position responsible for overseeing implementation of the plan of action.
- Although the PPR tool allows for only one person to be designated, you should also consider all staff who will be involved in implementation. Who is involved will depend on your organization, the standard, and the plan of action; however, it is important to consider involving direct care staff, leadership, and physicians (if applicable at your organization). For instance, your hospital or ambulatory surgery center or office-based surgery site might find that it has been noncompliant in implementing the recommendations associated with National Patient Safety Goal 4 that deals with eliminating wrong-site, wrong-patient, and wrong-procedure surgery. Staff involved in this example might include the medical director, medical staff, risk manager, anesthesia care providers, quality improvement, clinical care, organization educators, clinical nurse specialists in surgical services, surgery operations manager, and clinical resource specialists in sur-

gical care. Your organization's board of trustees, which also must make patient safety a priority, might also be included by being briefed on the plan of action and by receiving regular updates at monthly meetings. A home care organization that, for example, finds noncompliance with infection control standards might involve all staff members who have responsibilities related to equipment use. This might involve staff who keep equipment clean before it is delivered to the patient and while it is being delivered to the patient. Staff who pick up the dirty equipment from patient homes also would be included, along with leaders who oversee the entire organization's infection control program. At a behavioral health care organization that uses medications, for example, noncompliance with standards related to properly and safely storing medications might require involvement from the medical director, medical staff, nursing, and quality improvement.

- The date by which the plan will be implemented. When establishing a time frame, remember that this date cannot be more than 6 months from the time the plan of action is approved in order to ensure a 12-month track record of compliance.
- The nature and scope of the compliance. Each EP that is identified as partial compliance or insufficient compliance should be addressed. The staff person creating a particular plan of action can outline the problems in a sentence or two. The more concise the problem description, the more space that can be used to outline the proposed corrections and measurements.
- How your organization will resolve the issue. Staff completing the plan of action can determine this element by asking the following questions:
    - What actions can bring the EP into compliance?
    - How will these actions bring the EP into compliance?

  These actions do not need to be complex or research supported, but they should fit the problem identified and be appropriate for your organization.
- How the proposed actions will be implemented
- An MOS that will show the standard in compliance (if required). An MOS is a measurable, objective criterion that shows that your organization has achieved and maintained compliance with an EP. An EP requires an MOS if there is an "Ⓜ" symbol next to it. Typically, an MOS is related to an audit that determines whether an action is effective and sustained. Staff creating your organization's plan of action can determine appropriate MOS by asking, "What measurable, objective criteria can show the EP is in compliance?" Appropriate data to use may include medical records, staff interviews, facility inspections, or performance improvement data—any data that show a track record of compliance. If possible, it is most efficient to use existing data sources for the MOS. The data used as an MOS must show at least a 90% compliance rate with the EP. For example, if your organization chooses to take a random sample of 25 medical records and

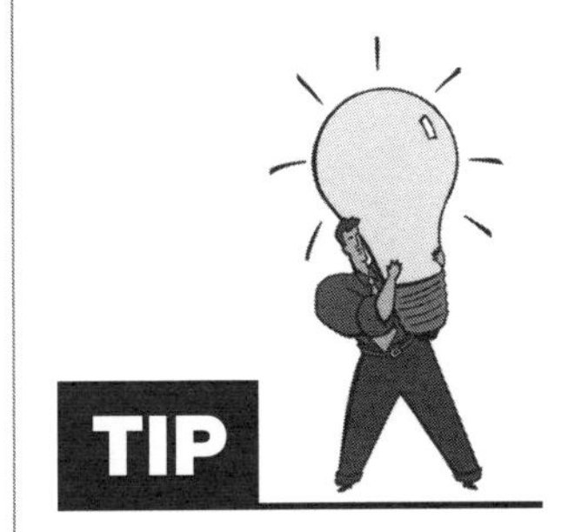

When implementing your organization's plan of action, ask staff to document how and when each planned action is being followed. For each action that is not being followed, determine why and whether modifications to the plan or additional education efforts are necessary.

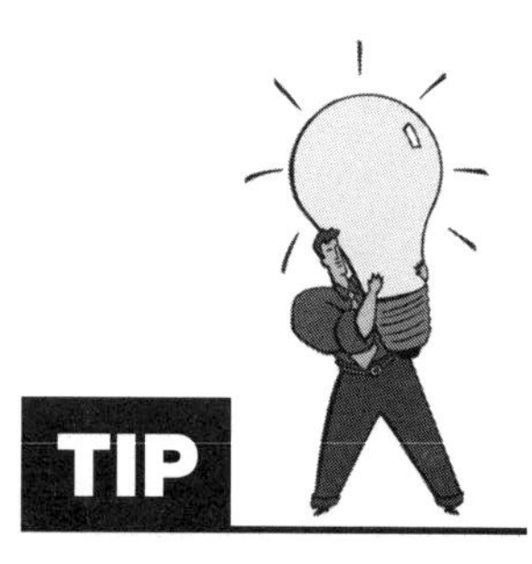

Only those standards identified as not compliant require a plan of action. However, staff may want to investigate and monitor compliant standards that have partially compliant EPs.

to use them as an MOS, then 90% of those records should reflect compliance with the EP.

In addition to these ideas, it may be helpful for your organization to identify how an EP was determined to be noncompliant or partially compliant. In other words, what data—medical records, interviews, facility tours, or performance improvement data—were used to come to the conclusion that your organization was noncompliant? This information can serve as a handy reference when staff develop MOS or begin to implement the plan of action.

It can also be helpful to identify possible causes of the compliance problem. For example, the causes may point to issues in allocating resources, lack of well-designed processes, or the need for leadership support. By identifying these possible causes, you may be able to reveal a larger problem that should be addressed. Several areas of noncompliance around a particular issue may point to a system or organization problem.

Educating Staff and Determining Staff Involved

Think of the plans of action as strategic priorities for your organization. These plans are "shared visions" that will lead your organization down "new pathways" to improvement. To meet the goals, though, you will need to build an atmosphere that makes these plans an organizationwide priority. Educating staff about the importance of the plans of action will help to accomplish this goal and offer staff motivation to complete what will become part of their everyday activities. See Sidebar 3-2 on page 39 for information on conducting a self-assessment to improve your plan of action.

Your staff members are likely already aware of problems and issues within your organization. The plan of action offers staff a constructive opportunity to address these issues in a positive, proactive way. The plan of action also provides an opportunity for staff to talk openly about problems and to come up with solutions without engaging in blame or recriminations. See Sidebar 3-3 on page 39 for information on the difference between a plan of action and an Evidence of Standards Compliance.

While the goals have been defined by the PPR process, the plan of action process offers your organization almost unlimited opportunities to involve staff in figuring out how to fix problems. Using a team approach in the plan of action allows various staff members to come together to create workable solutions, rather than, for example, carrying out a mandate from leadership. Staff can be creative in looking at the problem and take pride in devising strategies for improving their jobs and, therefore, the services your organization provides. Staff can develop plans of action that are most meaningful to your organization's unique characteristics.

Your organization may want to involve staff by appointing "champions" or someone who will be accountable for creating, implementing, and monitoring each of the plans. Keeping the approach to plans of action as simple and suc-

Sidebar 3-2: Using a Self-Assessment to Improve Your Plan of Action

To make sure that plans of action are actually being carried out, your organization may want to periodically conduct a self-assessment on those areas. You will be able to determine if a plan is being implemented and if performance is improving—the ultimate goal. If your assessment reveals that a plan is neither progressing nor producing the desired results, your organization can refocus its education efforts. However, if the assessment shows that your plan is on track and that improvement is being realized and sustained, then you have the "evidence" of successful implementation that will lead to improved quality and safety of care.

Sidebar 3-3: Difference Between a Plan of Action and an Evidence of Standards Compliance

To accomplish your organization's goals, be sure that staff directly involved in the accreditation process understand the difference between a plan of action and an Evidence of Standards Compliance report (ESC report). The plan of action is a strategy your organization will use to come into compliance with standards at the time of the PPR. The ESC report is an account of what has already been done to come into compliance after survey.

In education efforts, consider using these more detailed descriptions of both activities:

Plan of action. Part of the PPR, a plan of action is required at the 18-month point of an organization's triennial survey. For every standard self-identified as out of compliance, an organization will develop and submit a plan of action addressing standards identified as "not compliant" and all related EPs that were scored partially compliant or noncompliant. The plan of action details the issue, the solution, the time frame, and an MOS (if required).

Evidence of Standards Compliance report (ESC report). Replacing the Written Progress Report, this report requires organizations to document compliance with a standard, to describe actions taken to achieve compliance, to identify how ongoing compliance will be identified, and to set a goal (as a percentage) for compliance in the form of an MOS. The ESC is required only if a standard is found not compliant at the time of the on-site survey. For more information on the ESC report, please see the "Shared Visions–New Pathways: The New JCAHO Accreditation Process" chapter of the most recent version of your accreditation manual.

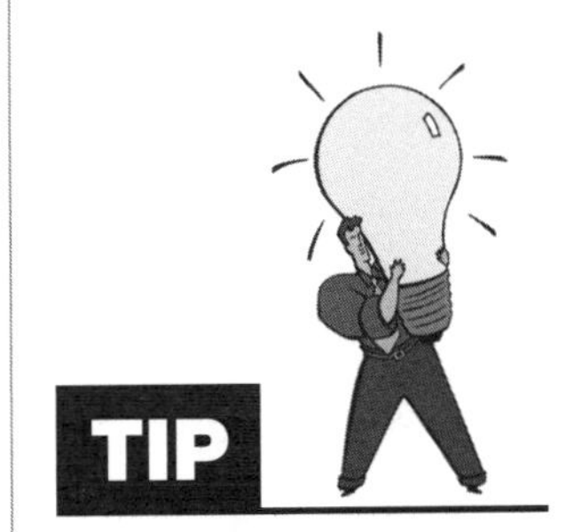

When creating a plan of action, determine whether a deficiency uncovered during your organization's self-assessment is specific to the area or is a systems problem appropriate for organizationwide improvement. Give staff involved in creating a plan of action approximately one to two weeks to complete this task.

cinct as possible is also a tactic that will help staff focus on the tasks. In addition, consider the "what" and "when" for each EP. "What" identifies how your organization plans to come into compliance with each EP that is noncompliant. "When" identifies time frames for implementing the plan. The 12-month track record necessary at the time of survey means that your organization should think in terms of an implementation time frame of 6 months or less, thus giving you plenty of time to put the actions into place.

Staff also might use the plan of action process as an opportunity to consider a few more facts. For example, looking at "where" the data came from may help uncover underlying systems issues. Asking the question "Why?" may help staff identify systems issues if several areas of noncompliance are found around a particular issue, such as staffing. Staff can then consider possible reasons for the noncompliance. For example, staffing issues may prompt those responsible for creating this particular plan of action to look at whether the number, competency, or qualifications of staff are affecting compliance. Or perhaps the problem stems from resource allocation issues such as training or inadequate monitoring of compliance with processes. Other areas to examine in tracing the cause of the issue might be lack of well-designed processes or leadership.

Choosing whom should be involved in creating and implementing the plan of action will depend on the standard addressed and the actions developed. At the very least, individuals involved with the issue should participate in the process. For example, physicians and other direct care providers, along with your organization's leaders, should be involved.

The plan of action can help your organization by more directly involving staff in the accreditation process. Because more than one staff member can access the automated PPR tool at the same time, the planning and implementing of improvements for several areas can occur simultaneously and in concert. For example, your organization may have one team working on infection control issues while another team handles noncompliance with a Management of Information standard.

This process also presents an ideal opportunity to involve groups not traditionally involved in standards evaluation (for example, information technology or physicians). In the examples of physicians and information technology, these particular staff members might generally recognize the importance of accreditation but in the past have not been easily able to identify areas where they could contribute to the process in a meaningful way. The PPR and its plan of action might supply that place, since they identify and solve systems problems.

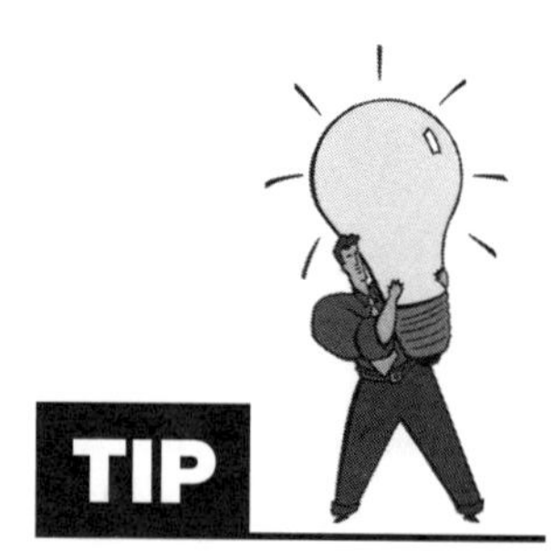

TIP

By involving staff in the PPR and plan of action, your organization makes them planners, data collectors, evaluators, and leaders. This self-discovery process enhances individual learning and can serve as a powerful vehicle for knowledge retention and staff buy-in.

When involving staff in the plan of action process, consider the following:

Education. Show staff members how this process will ultimately affect and improve the care they personally provide or the organization as a whole provides. Sharing information in an interactive format allows for questions, explanations, and discussion that helps staff to be active participants in the process. For example, education for physicians might include presentations at medical staff meetings or key medical/surgical department meetings. This plan presents an opportunity to demonstrate how important their involvement will be to the success of the plan of action.

Engagement. Give staff members a reason why they should want to be involved. For example, the plan of action will improve the care nurses deliver to their patients, residents, or clients. Your organization should also let staff members know their expected roles and activities, in addition to requesting specific time commitments while remaining sensitive to schedules and workloads. Ask staff experienced with the process or interested in a particular topic to be champions to stimulate interest among colleagues.

Empowerment. Focus staff time on systems and processes in which their input can make the biggest difference. Staff members will be more interested in participating if they think they can personally make a difference in the quality and safety of care provided by your organization.

The plan of action can also bring specific problems to the attention of staff members by taking them out of the realm of "JCAHO issues" that leaders must contend with into the realm of problems they can solve. Meaning less guesswork for front-line staff members who can now clearly understand how their daily work contributes to better care.

The PPR tool and plan of action also help leadership and supervisors by focusing their efforts. Supervisors, for example, can make a compelling case to leaders for investing time and resources to improve noncompliant areas. Or leaders can use the plan of action as a tool to guide improvement and education efforts more effectively. By focusing on measurable objectives, your organization can reinforce the idea of a systems approach to providing safe, high-quality care for patients that involves working across disciplines and departments in order to achieve your goals.

Finally, it will be important to remind staff members frequently that they do make a difference and that your organization cannot carry out its plan of action without them. See Sidebar 3-4 on page 45 for ideas on how staff can help identify compliance issues.

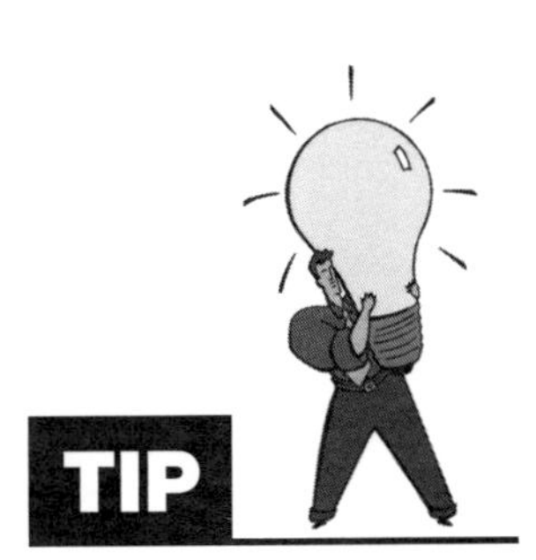

Ask staff to identify trouble spots in your organization. Determine how each trouble spot affects the quality and safety of care, treatment, and services and then identify solutions and methods to measure the effectiveness of proposed solutions. This exercise can be done throughout the accreditation cycle, not just at the midpoint or full survey time frame. Creating a simple compliance-issues log that identifies the functional area from the accreditation manual (for example, Management of Human Resources), the deficiency, and whether the issue is specific to an area or is organizationwide can then serve as a reference.

Sample Plan of Action: 1

Standard

Protocols for restraint use contain criteria to ensure only clinical justified use.

Element of Performance Out of Compliance

A licensed independent practitioner (LIP) issues a patient-specific order authorizing the use of restraint protocols.

Organization Findings

A random sample of medical records revealed that three of seven records reviewed in which restraint use was reflected did not have an order from an LIP authorizing the use of restraint protocols. None of the three absent orders originated from the same patient unit.

Plan of Action

Hospital policy regarding the use of restraints according to protocols and the requirement of an order from an LIP will be communicated to two targeted groups: medical staff members and nursing staff. Multiple vehicles will be used for this communication, including monthly medical staff meetings, clinical service meetings, nursing meetings, weekly Safety-Alert e-mails, and posted notices at nursing stations. Orientation and in-service curricula will be reviewed to ensure that the restraint policy is covered.

Method

By January 1, 2005, a representative sample of medical records will be audited by the hospital to ascertain whether restraint use authorized through protocols includes an order from an LIP.

Measure of Success

90% of audited records in compliance.

Sample Plan of Action: 2

Standard

The organization defines in writing the data and information gathered during assessment and reassessment.

EPs

A 1. The organization's written definition of the data and information gathered during assessment and reassessment include the following:

- The scope of assessment and reassessment activities by each discipline
- The content of the assessment and reassessment
- The criteria for when an additional or more in-depth assessment is done

A 2. The screening, assessment, and reassessment activities described are within the scope of practice, state licensure laws, applicable regulations, or certification of the discipline doing the assessment

B 3. If applicable, separate specialized assessment and reassessment information is identified for the various populations served

Areas of Noncompliance

Organization does not define in writing the criteria for when an additional or more in-depth assessment is done.

This issue was identified through interviews with staff members during tracers and a review of the assessment policy. There is a lack of clear policy required to initiate an additional or more in-depth assessment.

Plan of Action

1. Meet with care nursing and medical staff to discuss the approach to assessment and reassessment in light of patient safety and quality of care
2. Develop and/or revise in writing the contents of a complete assessment and reassessment
3. Revise the assessment form to more clearly include the criteria for performing additional or more in-depth assessments
4. Review and revise the policy on additional or more in-depth assessments, as necessary
5. Conduct an in-service about performing additional or more in-depth assessments

Due Date

5/22/04

Responsible Individual

Mary Smith, M.S.N.

MOS

Monthly audit of patient records indicating that 90% or more of all patients are checked against the criteria for reassessment or more in-depth assessment.

Sample Plan of Action: 3

During ABC Behavioral Health's PPR, the organization scored a restraint use standard as noncompliant.

Standard

The initial assessment of each individual at the time of admission or intake assists in obtaining information about the individual that could help minimize the use of restraint or seclusion.

EPs

The initial assessment of an individual who is at risk of harming himself or herself, or others, including staff identifies the following:

- Pre-existing medical conditions or any physical disabilities and limitations that would place the individual at greater risk during restraint or seclusion
- Any history of sexual or physical abuse that would place the individual at greater psychological risk during restraint or seclusion

Areas of Noncompliance

ABC Behavioral Health's initial assessment does not thoroughly address conditions or disabilities or history of physical abuse that might place the patient at greater risk for restraint/seclusion use.

This issue was identified through a review of records in the behavioral health unit. The sources of this situation appear to be a lack of clear policy, incomplete assessment forms, and inadequate communication/education about the assessment process.

Plan of Action

- Review and revise as necessary the policy on initial assessment
- Revise the assessment form
- Conduct in-service about initial assessment

Due Date

6/1/04

Responsible Individual

Restraint use monitor (nurse executive)

MOS

Monthly audit of patient records demonstrating that 90% or more of the records reviewed contain adequate information.

Sidebar 3-4: Identifying Compliance Issues

Your organization's JCAHO coordinator and members of the planning or performance improvement team may want to brainstorm a compliance plan for identified trouble spots. The plan can be documented and shared with all appropriate staff and departments, with a time line created for implementing the improvements. It may also be useful to prioritize the improvements. Allow one to two weeks for this process, depending on the results and complexity of the project.

To ensure success, do the following:

- Consider multivoting to reach consensus about actions that should be implemented for problems
- Identify benchmarks or performance indicators by which improvements will be measured
- Create a review schedule to monitor the process, ask for feedback on the plan from staff members involved in the affected processes, and allow time to make changes
- Create a simple compliance plan to record the standard number, EP, issue, action, MOS, committee member or staff responsible, target date, and completion date
- Make certain that each agreed-upon compliance plan includes baseline indicators and targets for successful implementation, or MOS, as required

CHAPTER FOUR

PRIORITY FOCUS PROCESS

The Priority Focus Process (PFP) is a part of the accreditation process that guides both the planning and conduct of your on-site survey. The PFP accomplishes these tasks by using information unique to your organization to more clearly focus the initial part of the on-site survey on areas most important to safety and quality of care. Essentially, the PFP is an internal JCAHO process that standardizes the review of data previously supplied to surveyors in raw form. Gathering data from multiple sources and analyzing the data using a defined, automated set of rules, the PFP turns these data into useful information.

JCAHO sought significant input from focus groups and conducted research to identify data associated with priority focus areas (PFAs) and to develop categories for sorting services provided and populations served, referred to as clinical/service groups (CSGs). A process was then identified to gather these data from multiple sources and to use automation to sort the data, formalizing the way presurvey information is used to guide the focus of the survey. See Sidebar 4-1 below for the definitions of PFA and CSG.

Sidebar 4-1: Priority Focus Areas and Clinical/Service Groups Definitions

Priority focus areas (PFAs) are processes, systems, or structures in a health care organization that can significantly impact the provision of safe, high-quality care and lead to positive outcomes when the process, system, or structure function properly.

Clinical/service groups (CSGs) are groups of patients in distinct, clinical populations for which data are collected. Tracer patients are selected according to CSGs.

Each PFA within the PFP is linked to revised standards. Using comprehensive, organization-specific data, the PFP identifies relevant standards for your organization's on-site survey. During the survey, surveyors will make connections between standards compliance issues and PFAs. When your organization is notified that it is time to select your Periodic Performance Review (PPR) option, you will receive a PFP summary that identifies PFAs and CSGs. This information provides a framework for your organization as you begin to assess compliance with standards but should not be limited to identified PFAs.

The changes to the survey process that are part of Shared Visions–New Pathways® are dependent upon the PFP because it will help organizations and surveyors make the most effective use of on-site survey time. The PFP provides this direction by centering the survey on care processes and systems important to your organization. By integrating information from the PFP to help focus the survey, the surveyor team starts to evaluate your organization. The identified CSGs point the surveyors toward the patient, resident, or client populations for tracer selection. The PFAs indicate what types of systems issues to look at during those visits.

An Overview of the Priority Focus Process

Both your organization and the surveyor team will receive access to your PFP information two weeks prior to the full survey. Your organization also will have received updated PFP information reflecting any new data received just prior to your PPR for your own reference. The PFP information will be used as follows:

- To convert presurvey data into information
- To focus survey activities
- As sampling criteria for the surveyors to select which type of patient, client, or resident to trace during the initial part of the survey
- To increase consistency in the survey process for organizations
- To customize the accreditation process to your unique organization

See Sidebar 4-2 on page 49 for information on types of data driving the Priority Focus Process.

PFAs serve as a framework in JCAHO's revised accreditation process, Shared Visions–New Pathways, by shaping the new on-site survey agenda. More important, your organization can use the PFA framework to continuously assess the strengths and weaknesses of your own essential processes and systems and to identify ways to enhance the provision of quality patient care in your organization.

PFAs are defined as processes, systems, or structures in a health care organization known to significantly impact safety and/or quality care. The PFAs were selected by JCAHO from a combination of sources—JCAHO's own internal databases, expert literature review, focus groups, and expert consensus. The PFAs

Sidebar 4-2: Type of Data Driving the Priority Focus Process

Internal JCAHO Data

- Prior accreditation history and recommendations
- Intracycle survey findings
- Quality Monitoring System data, including sentinel events and complaint history (received from patients, family members, staff, media reports, and so forth)
- Performance measurement data
- Data supplied by the health care organization in its electronic application for accreditation, including type and number of services, ownership, merger/acquisition information

External Data

- State agency communications
- Centers for Medicare & Medicaid Services data such as Medicare Provider Analysis and Review (MedPAR) for hospitals, including the following:
    - Full-time equivalent staff positions per average occupied beds
    - Volume per clinical/service group (CSG)
    - Average length of stay per CSG
    - Mortality rates per CSG
    - Complication rate per CSG
    - Medicare case mix index
    - Medicare utilization percentage

emerged after identifying common patterns constructive in building positive health care outcomes and enhancing the provision of safe, quality health care. The various processes, systems, and structures leading to improved health care were categorized into 15 PFAs. The 15 PFAs are as follows:

1. Assessment and Care/Services (not applicable for laboratories)
2. Communication
3. Credentialed Practitioners
4. Equipment Use
5. Infection Control
6. Information Management
7. Medication Management (not applicable for laboratories)
8. Organizational Structure
9. Orientation and Training
10. Rights and Ethics
11. Physical Environment
12. Quality Improvement Expertise and Activity
13. Patient Safety

14. Staffing
15. Analytical Procedures (replaces Assessment and Care/Services for laboratories only)

Educating Staff and Determining Staff Involved

In educating staff about the PFP, it is important to note that the new process is simply an automated decision support system that reviews presurvey materials consistently across all health care organizations yet keeps each review relevant to each specific organization. JCAHO has used a rules-based approach for years to determine survey complement, length, fee, and applicable standards manuals based on an organization's application for accreditation. PFP uses a similar rules-based system and can be thought of simply as sources of information that surveyors use to obtain data.

Staff involved in the accreditation process should understand that the data components used in the PFP include information from the Centers for Medicare & Medicaid Services (CMS) and ORYX® core measure data, complaint data, accreditation history data, and data provided by your organization in the application for accreditation. The PFP integrates these various presurvey data and recommends consistent areas of priority focus. Types of data fed into the PFP's automated tool include the following:

- Previous survey findings or recommendations, proficiency testing results (for laboratories), and ORYX® core measure data (if applicable)
- Data from JCAHO's Office of Quality Monitoring about your organization and data from your application for accreditation
- External data, such as Medicare Provider Analysis and Review (MedPAR) data

Not all accreditation programs will initially have external data sources to feed into the PFP. Behavioral health care and ambulatory care do not have organized data available at present. In addition, Veterans Administration, Shriner's, Children's, and military hospitals do not have MedPAR data as do other hospital organizations. Home care and long term care PFP data may include the use of CMS data in the future. Until the data can be obtained directly from CMS, JCAHO is pilot testing the use of data from Home Health Care Compare (populated with OASIS [Outcome and Assessment Information Set] data) and from Nursing Home Compare (populated with Minimum Data Set [MDS]) data, which are available at http://www.medicare.gov. OASIS is a key component of Medicare's partnership with the home care industry to foster and monitor improved home health care outcomes. Data items for home care encompass sociodemographic, environmental, support system, health status, functional status attributes of adult (nonmaternity) patients, and selected attributes of health service utilization. The MDS, which drives individualized care plans, is a mandated, standardized, comprehensive assessment of a long term care resident's functional, medical, psychosocial, and cognitive status. MDS information is collected and used to ensure that nursing home residents receive quality care and services in a safe and comfortable environment in accordance with rules established by CMS.

Two weeks before your organization's full survey, your staff and your assigned surveyors will have access to the PFP information through the extranet. This information will give the surveyor time to become familiar with your organization, the services it provides, and issues that are most relevant in assessing safety and quality. Specifically, surveyors will have the following information about your organization:

- Demographics
- The top four specific PFAs
- The top priority CSGs
- Standards associated with the PFAs

The top PFAs may be used in all survey activities. Information from prioritized PFAs and CSGs can help guide and focus other survey activities such as the following:

- Leadership Conference
- System Tracers
- Review of the Environment of Care
- Competency Assessment Process
- Individual tracers

Not all of these activities, however, apply to all settings.

Your organization can use information about your PFAs to continuously assess the strengths and weaknesses of essential processes and systems. This plan can in turn guide education efforts and help you identify ways to enhance the provision of quality care.

Your organization can use PFA information to plan education for staff on both a formal and informal basis. For example, an in-service training program might focus on infection control. In this example, the session, which could be adjusted to meet the needs of various disciplines or departments, would include the following:

- Review of the infection control program, including an emphasis on the importance of infection control, your organization's commitment to infection control, and leadership and staff accountabilities for infection control
- Review of your infection control practices, including instructions on surveillance, data collection, terminology, and so forth
- Implementation of infection control policies, procedures, and tools, including the relationship to JCAHO standards
- Information on how staff members play a role in infection control

- Information about where staff can easily access your organization's infection control guidelines, along with expert literature
- Discussion of infection control performance improvement efforts, including measures and goals
- Question-and-answer period

Sample Priority Focus Process Summary

Memorial General Hospital
Priority Focus Process Information—January 2004

Overview

The Priority Focus Process (PFP) is a component of Shared Visions–New Pathways, a new accreditation process introduced by JCAHO in 2004. The PFP consistently uses presurvey information about health care organizations to create priorities for reviewing standards compliance, thus lending consistency to the survey process. The results for your organization are listed below.

Priority Focus Areas

Priority focus areas (PFPs) are processes, systems, or structures in a health care organization that significantly impact the quality and safety of care. Your organization's prioritized PFAs (and definitions for those areas) are as follows:

Assessment and Care/Services

Assessment and care/services for individuals comprise a series of processes, including, as relevant, assessment; planning care, treatment, and/or services; provision of care; ongoing reassessment of care; and discharge planning, referral for continuing care, or discontinuation of services. Assessment and care/services are fluid in nature to accommodate a patient's needs while in a care setting. Although some elements of assessment and care/services may occur only once, other aspects may be repeated or revisited as the patient's needs or care delivery priorities change. Successful implementation of improvement in assessment and care/services relies on the full support of leadership.

Communication

Communication is the process by which information is exchanged between individuals, departments, or organizations. Effective communication successfully permeates every aspect of a health care organization from the provision of care to performance improvement, resulting in a marked improvement in the quality of care delivery and functions. Subprocesses for communication include the following:

- Provider and/or staff-patient communication
- Patient and family education
- Staff communication and collaboration
- Information dissemination
- Multidisciplinary teamwork

continued on page 53

Sample Priority Focus Process Summary *(continued from page 52)*

Information Management

Information Management is the interdisciplinary field concerning the timely and accurate creation, collection, storage, retrieval, transmission, analysis, control, dissemination, and use of data or information both within an organization and externally, as allowed by law and regulation. In addition to written and verbal information, supporting information technology and information services are also included in Information Management. Subprocesses for Information Management include the following:

- Planning
- Procurement
- Implementation
- Collection
- Recording
- Protection
- Aggregation
- Interpretation
- Storage and retrieval
- Data integrity
- Information dissemination

Organizational Structure

The Organizational Structure is the framework for an organization to carry out its vision and mission. The implementation is accomplished through corporate bylaws and governing body policies, organization management, compliance, planning, integration and coordination, and performance improvement. Included are the organization's governance, business ethics, contracted organizations, and management requirements. Subprocesses for Organizational Structure include the following:

- Management requirements
- Corporate bylaws and governing body plans
- Organization management
- Compliance
- Planning
- Business ethics
- Contracted services

Clinical/Service Groups

Clinical/service groups CSGs are categories of patients or services at a health care organization for which data are collected. Your hospital's prioritized CSGs (and types of patients included in these groups) are as follows:

General Surgery
Appendectomy, hernia repairs, rectal resection, peritoneal adhesiolysis, small and large bowel procedures, stomach/esophageal/duodenal procedures, pancreas, liver and shunt procedures,

continued on page 54

Sample Priority Focus Process Summary *(continued from page 53)*

biliary tract procedures, cholecystectomy (nonlaparoscopic), mastectomy, skin graft/debridement, wound debridement for injuries, amputation of lower limb, adrenal and pituitary procedures, thyroid and parathyroid procedures, other endocrine procedure, lymphoma, leukemia with procedure, male reproductive system procedure, splenectomy, hand procedures, breast procedure for nonmalignancy, and outpatient services, including general surgery, pain management, plastic surgery, and outpatient surgery

Thoracic Surgery
Major chest procedures, respiratory system surgical procedures, major chest trauma, and lung transplant

Dermatology
Pressure ulcers, skin disorders, nonmalignant breast disorders, cellulites, trauma to skin, subcutaneous tissue, and breast

Neurosurgery
Craniotomy, spinal procedures, carpal tunnel release, peripheral and cranial nerve procedures, traumatic stupor and coma, anterior/posterior spinal fusion, spinal fusion, and back and neck procedures

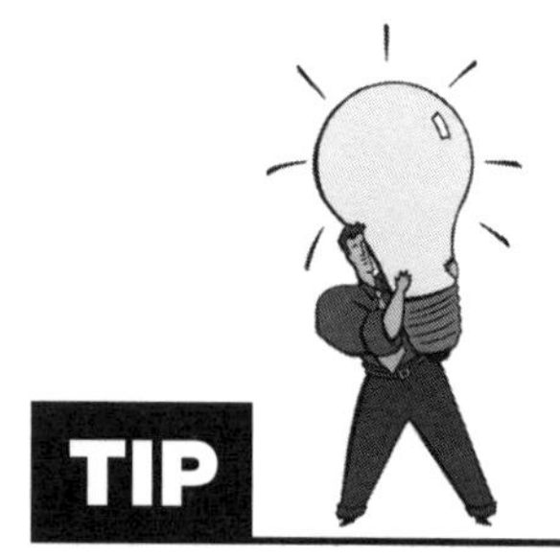

Ask staff members to think about how their knowledge and experience contributes to safety and quality as they apply to each PFA and CSG.

Clinical/Service Groups

Clinical/service groups (CSGs) categorize patients into distinct populations on which JCAHO can gather data to help create an individualized picture of your organization. Individuals chosen for initial tracer activities during your on-site survey are selected according to your CSGs. See Table 4-1 on page 55 for CSGs by accreditation program.

Table 4-1: Priority Focus Process Output

Clinical/Service Groups by Accreditation Program		
AMBULATORY HEALTH CARE *Medical/Dental* Cardiology Dentistry Dermatology Emergency medicine Family practice Gastroenterology General practice Internal medicine Neurology Obstetrics/gynecology Occupational health Oncology Optometry Orthopedic medicine Otolaryngology Pediatric medicine Pharmacy/dispensary Podiatry	Rheumatology Short stay/observation/infirmary/recovery Urology Vascular medicine *Surgery/Anesthesia* Cardiac catheterization Endoscopy Gastroenterology procedures General surgery In vitro fertilization Ophthalmology Oral maxillofacial surgery Orthopedic surgery Plastic surgery Podiatric surgery Trigger point injections (pain management) Urologic procedures	*Diagnostic/Therapeutic Services/Other* Allergy Alternative/complementary care Audiology Chiropractic medicine Diagnostic imaging Dialysis Hematology Infusion therapy Lithotripsy Orthotics/prosthetics Pain management Physical medicine and rehabilitation Pulmonary medicine Radiation oncology Sleep diagnostics Waived laboratory testing Other
ASSISTED LIVING Activities/socialization Contracted health care services Hospitality support services In-house nursing care services Medication services	Specialty service—dementia Specialty service—children/young adults Specialty service—neurologic/TBI Specialty service—HIV	Specialty service—cosmetic surgery recovery Specialty service—hospice Specialty service—wound care Specialty service—rehabilitation Specialty service—other
BEHAVIORAL HEALTH CARE * Adult day care Assertive community treatment Behavioral health services Case management Chemical dependency	Correctional behavioral health Developmental disabilities Family preservation/wraparound services Forensic behavioral health Foster care In-home behavioral health Methadone detoxification	Methadone maintenance Outdoor behavioral health Post-acute acquired brain injury Shelter Therapeutic foster care Vocational rehabilitation

* Applies to both child and adult populations

continued on page 56

Priority Focus Process Output *(continued from page 55)*

CRITICAL ACCESS HOSPITAL

Cardiology (core measure)*
Dentistry
Dermatology
Endocrinology
Gastroenterology
General medicine
General surgery
Gynecology
Hematology
HIV infection
Neonatology (core measure)
Nephrology
Normal newborns
Obstetrics (core measure)
Oncology
Ophthalmology
Orthopedics
Otolaryngology
Pediatrics (core measure)
Psychiatry
Pulmonary (core measure)
Rehabilitation
Rheumatology
Substance abuse
Thoracic surgery
Trauma
Urology
Vascular surgery
Other

HEALTH CARE NETWORK

Heath Maintenance Organization (HMO)
Integrated Delivery Network (IDN)
Managed behavioral health care organization
Continuing care services
Specialty care—behavioral health
Specialty care—physical therapy
Specialty care—pharmacy
Specialty care—podiatric
Specialty care—surgical/subspecialty
Specialty care—chiropractic
Specialty care—eye care
Specialty care—dental
Specialty care—pediatric
Other

HOME CARE

Home Medical Equipment

HME–Clinical respiratory services
HME–Home medical equipment services
HME–Rehabilitation technology

Hospice

HOS–Facility-based respite care
HOS–Facility-based symptom relief
HOS–Hospice in-home care

Pharmacy

RX–Clinical consultant pharmacist
RX–Freestanding ambulatory infusion
RX–Long term care pharmacy dispensing
RX–Pharmacy dispensing

Home Health

HH–Home health services
HH–Home personal care/support services

Additional Home Health Based on CMS' Home Health Care Compare Data

HH–Patients having acute care hospitalizations
HH–Patients having confusion difficulties
HH–Patients having emergent care
HH–Patients having pain interfering with activity
HH–Patients needing ambulation improvement
HH–Patients needing bathing assistance
HH–Patients needing oral medication management
HH–Patients needing toileting assistance
HH–Patients needing transferring assistance
HH–Patients needing upper body dressing assistance

---

* As of July 1, 2002, hospitals are required to collect data on two of the four core measures identified in this list and to submit that data through a listed performance measurement system by January 31, 2003.

continued on page 57

Priority Focus Process Output *(continued from page 56)*

HOSPITAL

Inpatient

Cardiac surgery
Cardiology (core measure)
Dentistry
Dermatology
Endocrinology
Gastroenterology
General medicine
General surgery
Gynecology
Hematology
HIV infection
Neonatology (core measure)
Nephrology
Neurology
Neurosurgery
Normal newborns
Obstetrics (core measure)
Oncology
Ophthalmology
Orthopedic
Other
Otolaryngology (core measure)
Pediatrics
Psychiatry
Pulmonary (core measure)
Rehabilitation
Rheumatology
Substance abuse
Thoracic surgery
Trauma
Urology
Vascular surgery

Laboratories

Blood donor center
Chemistry
Clinical cytogenetics immunogenetics
Diagnostic immunology
Embryology
Hematology
Histocompatibility
Immunohematology
Microbiology
Molecular biology
Pathology
PPMP* testing services
Radiobioassay
Tissue storage
Waived services

LONG TERM CARE

Long Term Care

LTC-Hospital operated
LTC-Freestanding
Residents needing subacute care

Additional LTC Based on CMS' Nursing Home Compare Data

Residents having delirium
Residents having infections
Residents having loss of ability in activities of daily living
Residents having mobility concerns
Residents having pressure ulcers
Residents needing pain control
Residents needing physical restraints

OFFICE-BASED SURGERY

Cardiac catheterization
Endoscopy
Gastroenterology procedures
General surgery
In vitro fertilization
Ophthalmology
Oral maxillofacial surgery
Orthopedic surgery
Plastic surgery
Podiatric surgery
Trigger point injections (pain management)
Urologic procedures

PREFERRED PROVIDER ORGANIZATION

Preferred Provider Organization
Other

---

* Provider-performed microscopic procedures

Sample Priority Focus Process Summary

The Priority Focus Process is a component of Shared Visions–New Pathways—the Joint Commission's accreditation process beginning January 2004. The Priority Focus Process consistently uses presurvey information about health care organizations to create priorities for reviewing standards compliance thus lending consistency to the survey process. Presurvey information is gleaned from data in your organization's application for accreditation, your organization's past survey findings, our Quality Monitoring System database of complaints and sentinel events, any ORYX® core measure data, and certain external data, if available. External data consist of publicly available data that are applicable to the accreditation program(s) being surveyed, such as MedPAR for hospitals, Nursing Home Compare, Home Health Compare, and failed laboratory proficiency testing data from CMS. The Priority Focus Process brings consistency to the survey process for organizations having similar presurvey data for the early part of their surveys as surveyors use the priority focus areas and clinical/service groups depicted in this report. However, based on initial findings, surveyors will broaden or change focus appropriately. Organizations performing their own standards compliance assessment for their Periodic Performance Review can use this information to enhance their evaluations, as well. The results for your organization are listed below.

XYZ Laboratory

Survey Date: July 7 – July 11, 2003
Event Type: Full Survey
PFT Updated: June 26, 2003

HCO ID: 999999
XYZ Hospital
1234 Street
City, State 99999

HCO Contact: Debbie Jones,
999-999-9999

Priority Focus Areas

Priority Focus Areas are defined as processes, systems, or structures in a health care organization that significantly impact the quality and safety of care.

Priority Focus Areas	Priority Clinical/Services Groups
Communication	Microbiology
Information Management	Pathology
Organizational Structure	Hematology
Analytical Procedures	Tissue Storage

Communication

Communication is the process by which information is exchanged between individuals, departments, or organizations. Effective communication successfully permeates every aspect of a health care organization from the provision of care to performance improvement, resulting in a marked improvement in the quality of care delivery and functioning.

continued on page 59

Sample Priority Focus Process Summary *(continued from page 58)*

Subprocesses for Communication include the following:

- Provider and/or staff-patient communication
- Patient and family education
- Staff communication and collaboration
- Information dissemination
- Multidisciplinary teamwork

LAB Standards that have been linked to Communication include the following:

APR 1	APR 8	EC.4.10	EC.9.20	IM.1.10	IM.6.180	LD.2.110	LD.3.50	PI.2.30
APR 10	APR 9	EC.5.20	EC.9.30	IM.2.10	IM.6.200	LD.2.120	LD.3.60	WT.1.10
APR 12	EC.1.10	EC.6.10	HR.1.10	IM.2.20	IM.6.260	LD.2.130	LD.4.10	WT.1.30
APR 2	EC.1.30	EC.7.10	IC.1.10@LAB	IM.3.10	LD.1.20	LD.2.160	LD.4.20	WT.1.40
APR 7	EC.3.10	EC.9.10	IC.3.10@LAB	IM.5.10	LD.2.100	LD.2.70	PI.1.10	

Information Management

Information management is the interdisciplinary field concerning the timely and accurate creation, collection, storage, retrieval, transmission, analysis, control, dissemination, and use of data or information both within an organization and externally, as allowed by law and regulation. In addition to written and verbal information, supporting information technology and information services are also included in information management.

Subprocesses for Information Management include the following:

- Planning
- Procurement
- Implementation
- Collection
- Recording
- Protection
- Aggregation
- Interpretation
- Storage and retrieval
- Data integrity
- Information dissemination

LAB Standards that have been linked to Information Management include the following:

APR 1	EC.3.10	EC.6.20	IM.1.10	IM.4.10	IM.6.210	IM.6.260	LD.2.160	LD.4.70	WT.1.30
APR 12	EC.4.10	EC.7.10	IM.2.10	IM.5.10	IM.6.220	LD.1.20	LD.2.200	PI.1.10	WT.1.40
APR 9	EC.5.10	EC.7.30	IM.2.20	IM.6.180	IM.6.230	LD.2.110	LD.2.70	PI.2.10	WT.1.60
EC.1.10	EC.5.40	EC.9.10	IM.2.30	IM.6.190	IM.6.240	LD.2.130	LD.3.50	PI.2.30	WT.1.30
EC.2.10	EC.6.10	HR.1.10	IM.3.10	IM.6.200	IM.6.250	LD.2.150	LD.4.60	PI.3.10	

continued on page 60

Sample Priority Focus Process Summary *(continued from page 59)*

Organizational Structure

The organizational structure is the framework for an organization to carry out its vision and mission. The implementation is accomplished through corporate bylaws and governing body polices, organization management, compliance, planning, integration and coordination, and performance improvement. Included are the organization's governance, business ethics, contracted organizations, and management requirements.

Subprocesses for Organizational Structure include the following:

- Management requirements
- Corporate bylaws and governing body plans
- Organization management
- Compliance
- Planning
- Business ethics
- Contracted services

LAB Standards that have been linked to Organizational Structure include the following:

APR 1	APR 3	EC.2.10	IC.1.10@LAB	IM.2.30	IM.6.250	LD.2.140	LD.2.140	LD.3.50	PI.2.30
APR 10	APR 7	EC.3.10	IC.3.10@LAB	IM.3.10	LD.1.10	LD.2.170	LD.2.170	LD.4.10	WT.1.10
APR 11	APR 8	EC.4.10	IM.1.10	IM.6.180	LD.1.20	LD.2.180	LD.2.180	LD.4.50	WT.1.20
APR 12	APR 9	EC.6.10	IM.2.10	IM.6.190	LD.1.30	LD.2.190	LD.2.190	LD.4.70	WT.1.40
APR 2	EC.1.10	EC.8.30	IM.2.20	IM.6.230	LD.2.110	LD.2.200	LD.2.200	PI.1.10	

Analytic Procedures

The laboratory's main function is that of conducting preanalytic, analytic, and postanalytic procedures.

Subprocesses for Analytic Procedures include the following:

- Request
- Specimen Collection
- Transportation
- Receipt
- Processing
- Testing
- Interpretation of Results
- Data Report/Dissemination

LAB Standards that have been linked to Analytic Procedures include the following:

EC.4.10	PI.1.10	WT.1.50
IM.4.10	PI.2.20	WT.1.60
IM.6.180	WT.1.10	
IM.6.190	WT.1.30	
IM.6.230	WT.1.40	

continued on page 61

Sample Priority Focus Process Summary *(continued from page 60)*

Clinical Service Groups

Clinical/Service Groups (CSGs) are categories of patients/residents/clients or services at a health care organization for which data are collected. They are not necessarily based on volume but are derived from several sources of data (that is, past survey recommendations, Joint Commission's complaint database, external sources such as Lab Proficiency Failures, and your organization's application for accreditation). These categories can be used for discussion in relation to priority focus areas (PFAs) and standards and to identify laboratory tests for additional focus in system level tracers. Types of tests that are included in your organization's top CSG categories are listed below:

Microbiology
Bacteriology, mycobacteriology, mycology, parasitology, virology

Pathology
Histopathology, oral pathology, dermatopathology, cytology

Hematology
Andrology, coagulation, hematology

Tissue Storage

CHAPTER FIVE

ON-SITE SURVEY PROCESS

When surveyors arrive at your organization for a full survey, all of the components of the Shared Visions–New Pathways® accreditation initiative will be put into action. The on-site survey has traditionally been a time of trepidation for many organizations, and the new process—including the start of unannounced surveys in 2006—is still likely to be a time of some nervousness. Education about the on-site process can help staff members feel more confident that they are ready individually and that the organization is ready as a whole to achieve accreditation. This education process builds upon all of the other learning experiences about the various components of accreditation. Staff members can also find satisfaction in knowing that their focus on continuous standards compliance means that your organization is doing its best to provide safe, quality care and is using the JCAHO standards as an operational guide.

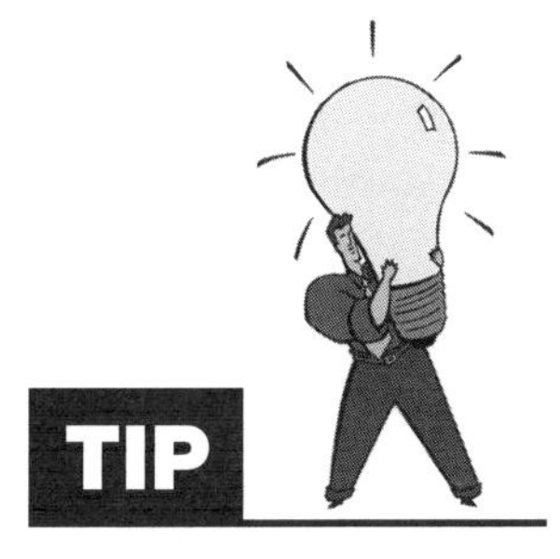

TIP

To create greater interest in learning about the on-site survey, consider asking staff what their goals are or asking them to set a particular goal for this process. Organizations that used scores as goals in the past will have to find new benchmarks now that scores have been eliminated. Instead, your organization might want to focus on being in full compliance with all standards all of the time. Other benchmarks for your organization might include staff and physician involvement in the accreditation process and satisfaction with that involvement.

An Overview of the On-Site Survey Process

The new survey process focuses on organization-specific, priority care processes and systems by incorporating information from the Priority Focus Process (PFP) to concentrate the survey on areas that are most critical to each health care organization's successful provision of safe, high-quality care. By adding a midcycle assessment of standards through the Periodic Performance Review (PPR), JCAHO moves health care organizations to a more continuous accreditation process—one that focuses on using the standards every day, 365 days a year, as an operational guide to providing safe, high-quality care. Along with the reformatting and clarifying of standards to focus more directly on safety, quality, and a new scoring and decision process, these elements of Shared Visions–New Pathways represent a complete paradigm shift from a process focused on survey preparation and score achievement to one of continuous systems and operational improvement. The culmination of these changes will be evident to your organization and its staff during the full on-site survey.

JCAHO will evaluate direct care by tracing the paths of patients, residents, or clients through your organization. A significant component of the new on-site process will include interaction with your organization's staff members in their units as JCAHO surveyors use the tracer methodology to follow the care of patients, clients, or residents through your units to see the direct provision of care, treatment, and services. More than ever before, surveyors will look at how your organization goes about providing care, treatment, and services on a daily basis.

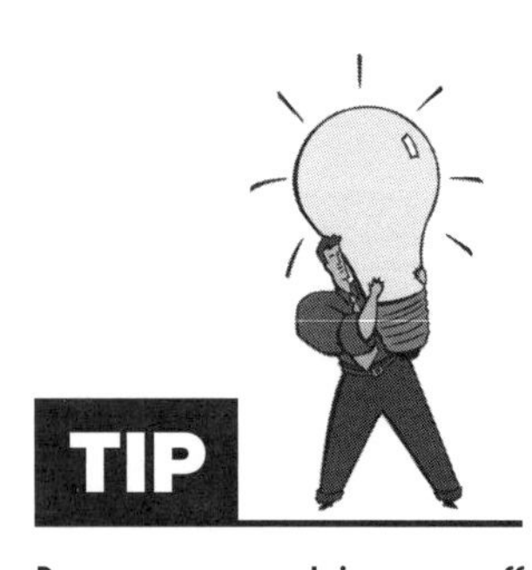

Be sure to explain to staff members that they do not need to know JCAHO standards; they just need to know their jobs. Surveyors talking with staff during the on-site survey are focusing on how staff would provide care in the tracer patient's situation. It is the surveyor's job to evaluate how the care provided relates to the concepts defined in JCAHO standards.

Educating Staff and Determining Staff Involved

Almost all staff should be prepared to be involved in the on-site survey process. Staff members could range from pharmacy at a long term care organization to housekeeping at a hospital. While surveys will move from announced to unannounced in 2006, it is a good idea to have staff stay aware of the process and be prepared during an accreditation year. See Sidebar 5-1 for ideas on helping staff understand the new survey process.

In addition to previous education efforts and an emphasis on continuous compliance with standards on a daily basis, your organization's staff members will be better prepared for the on-site survey if they understand the various components of the process. The new on-site survey agenda is designed to be in line with your organization's normal operational systems. This agenda will mean fewer formal interviews, such as surveyors and leaders or supervisors sitting in a conference room. The formal document review session, for example, has been eliminated, along with prescheduled visits to care settings and functional interviews. In the past, for example, surveyors may have talked with leaders, physicians, and staff at a hospital about policies, education, and other steps they took to prevent wrong-site surgery. Now, surveyors will look at a hospital's efforts by tracing a patient through the organization, from the time of admission until the time of discharge, to gather information.

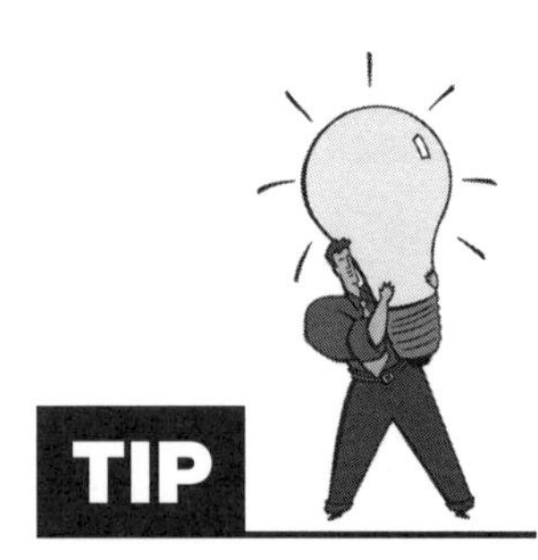

An important goal of the revised survey process is to better engage direct care providers in the accreditation process. The process also encourages multilevel participation of leaders and staff.

While some of the more formal, preplanned aspects of the survey have been eliminated, your organization's JCAHO coordinator or performance improvement director will still want to plan for the on-site visit and help staff learn about how the process will be conducted. Your organization's JCAHO coordinator or performance improvement director may want to review the finalized survey agenda and priority focus areas (PFAs) with involved staff. It may also be useful to share the list of the main PFAs to be addressed during the survey with all staff. This finalized agenda will be delivered to both your organization and the assigned surveyors about 14 days before the anticipated site visit, along with the PFP output. This output identifies the top four PFAs and clinical/service groups (CSGs) that will be the focus of the visit and helps determine the surveyors' selection of charts and other records to trace.

In addition, your organization may want to consider conducting a walk-through of the site visit with each section supervisor or manager. The JCAHO coordinator and performance improvement team leaders can conduct a run-

Sidebar 5-1: Helping Staff Understand the New Survey Process

To help staff understand how the on-site survey process works and to be thoroughly prepared to make the most of your organization's accreditation efforts, it may be useful to create a schedule. This schedule could, for example, list what your organization needs to accomplish to be ready for the on-site survey. This might start with preparations such as creating multidisciplinary teams to carry out plans of action, conduct mock surveys, and communicate with colleagues about the process. Or, your organization may choose to conduct a SWOT (Strengths, Weaknesses, Opportunities, and Threats) analysis on the on-site survey process. Listing time frames, tasks, and accountabilities will help to ensure that your organization meets its goals.

through of the visit with each supervisor to familiarize him or her with the events that are likely to occur. It may also be helpful to consider any problems that may occur prior to or during the survey (for example, job actions or other union activity, or the absence of a particular director or administrative representative during your survey). By listing any potential problems, staff can identify alternative leaders, or communication techniques.

In addition, keep in mind that all site visits will be unannounced beginning in 2006. This change should present no problem for your organization, assuming that staff members have kept up with the tasks listed below, which are designed to help you maintain a state of continuous standards compliance. Typically, the JCAHO coordinator and members of your organization's performance improvement team will be responsible for working with staff members to educate them about how to accomplish these tasks. Your organization can maintain continuous standards compliance by performing some or all of the following tasks:

- Share information with all staff about the change from the triennial survey to the unannounced survey beginning in 2006
- Seek out peer institutions against which to benchmark your performance
- Be aware of the possibility of unannounced surveys beginning in 2006
- Read *Joint Commission Perspectives®* newsletter to keep abreast of standards changes as they occur
- Visit the JCAHO Web site regularly to keep current with standards-related changes and initiatives
- Maintain a track record of your compliance with all standards (not an accreditation requirement)
- Ensure that your organization is maintaining a track record of compliance with the National Patient Safety Goals and their requirements for current and past years, and stay aware of the results
- Begin to plan for new standard implementation as soon as such standards are published
- Inform relevant staff members about any new standards and educate staff

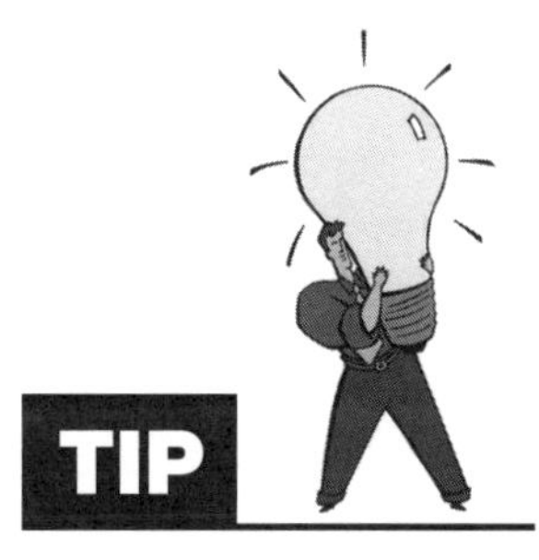

Help staff members prepare for interaction with JCAHO surveyors by emphasizing that they are the "experts" when it comes to their individual duties. Surveyors simply want to know how staff deliver care, treatment, or services; staff are not expected to recite standards. Staff asked a question by a surveyor should carefully listen to the question, and answer honestly.

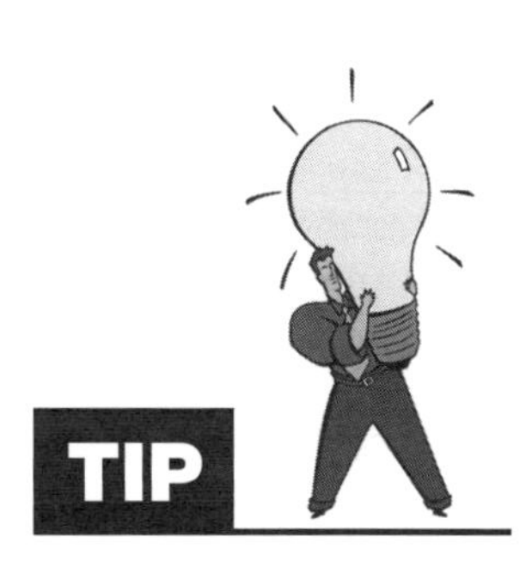

Encourage staff to think of the on-site survey as an opportunity for professional development. Staff can use interactions with surveyors to learn how other organizations address similar issues and to plan for future improvement opportunities by making note of comments by surveyors.

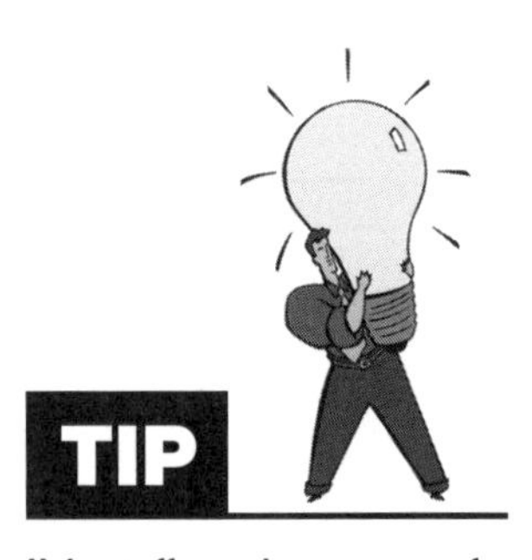

Help staff members prepare for interaction with surveyors and feel more comfortable with their knowledge by randomly posing sample questions during the months leading up to the on-site survey. For example, your organization's designated JCAHO coordinator may want to ask a member of the medical records staff how he or she ensures that summary lists for a particular patient are up-to-date. Or a variety of staff could be asked about the process they use for the read-back of verbal orders. Physicians might be asked how they are involved in improving patient safety. Supervisors or department managers could also conduct these activities.

members on how to comply with the new standards as part of their daily work routine

- Start tracking compliance with new standards the day they take effect
- Schedule staff to attend education programs offered by Joint Commission Resources and state associations
- Schedule and conduct mock surveys regularly
- Provide in-services to educate staff about new systems
- Make performance improvement a top priority

Every survey will be as unique as the organizations involved, but here is a brief summary of the activities during the full on-site survey so that staff can know what to expect and who will be involved. This list can help your organization direct education efforts.

Opening Conference and Orientation. This first element of the survey allows for introductions among key organization staff and the surveyors. Your organization will provide information about its purpose and structure to help guide the surveyors. This presentation should not be elaborate or lengthy, but all services provided should be addressed. Your organization's surveyors will briefly describe the structure of the survey and remind you of the data and information needed to complete the next element of the survey, which is the survey planning session.

Senior leadership should attend this session to discuss their responsibilities in your organization for planning, management, oversight, performance improvement, and support in carrying out the mission and strategic objectives. Leaders will be asked to talk about your organization's strategic planning and resource allocation and how performance improvement expectations are established, planned, prioritized, and managed. Although the structure of your organization, along with the care and services provided, will determine who is involved in the opening conference and orientation, typically at least one member of the governing body or a trustee participates. This individual may be the CEO if your organization has a single owner. Senior organization leaders, such as the CEO, COO, CIO, nurse executive, laboratory medical director, director of patient or client services, and so forth also should expect to participate in this session.

Surveyor Planning Session. During this session, the surveyors will review the data and information about your organization and plan the direction of the survey. The surveyors will select initial tracer patients, clients, or residents by reviewing your top PFAs and CSGs to identify areas of care, treatment, and service and patient populations that are priorities for your facility. If your organization has more than one surveyor assigned to the survey, the surveyors will coordinate tracer activities so that no more than one surveyor will visit the same unit in your organization at the same time or need to speak to the same staff members at the same time. Surveyors will review achievement of measures of success (MOS) contained in the plan of action from your organization's PPR activities.

Surveyors may call upon your organization's JCAHO coordinator during this session if they have questions. In addition, staff knowledgeable about current active patients, residents, or clients may be requested to assist your surveyors in identifying initial tracer individuals.

Individual Tracer Activity. The tracer methodology will drive the majority of the new survey process at your organization. The tracer methodology is a way to analyze your organization's systems of providing care, treatment, and services using actual care recipients as the framework for assessing standards compliance. On the first day of your survey, the survey team will select individuals to use in the tracer process based on the following criteria (as applicable to your organization):

- Care recipients from the top CSGs identified in your PFP Summary Report, which will be available on your extranet site two weeks before your survey
- Individuals whose care experience has taken them through areas that are a part of system tracers (infection control, data use, and medication management)
- Individuals who cross programs (for example, a patient who has undergone diagnostic testing at an ambulatory facility, had surgery in a hospital, and been discharged to a rehabilitation center or home care)
- Individuals who have received care, treatment, or services in multiple areas of your organization

These are only some of the initial considerations for tracer selection, but findings from other survey activities may suggest additional parameters. Surveyors will give your organization a list of these criteria and ask staff to pull care recipient records that fit these criteria. See Sidebar 5-2 for additional information on individual tracers.

Sidebar 5-2: Understanding the Individual Tracer

When educating staff about the individual tracer activity, questions may come up about how this applies to long term care, ambulatory care, or home care settings in which the patient does not physically move within the organization or there is not a variety of services provided. The answer is that JCAHO surveyors are not tracing the geography of your organization but the variety of care, treatment, and services provided to an individual, even if that care is provided in a single room or in a home setting. For example, if a long term care resident's chart indicates that he is receiving pharmacy services or a nutritional assessment at the current location, the surveyor will know that medication management and nutrition systems are involved in caring for this particular resident. The surveyor will visit the pharmacy and dietary services to speak with staff about this particular resident.

Once individual tracers are identified for your facility, surveyors will follow or "trace" the care provided to an individual by following how that care was provided throughout your organization to specific patients, residents, or clients. For most organizations, surveyors will start where the care recipient is currently located. They can then move to where the patient, client, or resident first entered your organization's systems, an area of care provided to the individual that may be a priority for your organization, or to any areas in your organization where the patient received care, treatment, or services. The order will vary because there is no specific order for visits to applicable care areas or departments. One approach is to follow the course of care received by the individual sequentially. Along the way, surveyors will speak with your organization's staff members who actually provided the care to that tracer individual—or, if that staff member is not available, surveyors will talk with another staff member who provides the same type of care. If a surveyor identifies a compliance issue, or if several surveyors on your team identify the same issue, the surveyors may pull additional records to identify if the issue is isolated or represents a bigger issue for your organization. Each tracer can take from an hour to three hours to complete. For example, a three-day survey may include an average of 11 individual tracers.

Any staff member at your organization could be part of this process ranging from human resource professionals to nurses to referral coordinators to home medical equipment drivers to receptionists to medical equipment managers to phlebotomists to environmental services staff.

To help staff understand the surveyors' use of tracer methodology, it may be useful prior to the on-site survey to randomly select individual results in a particular area (ventilator care, for example, at a home care organization) and trace the patient through his or her entire care experience. Or, for example, surveyors might select a patient admitted to a hospital's emergency department with pain from a pressure ulcer. The surveyor would look at the patient's care in the emergency, radiology, and surgery departments, along with any nutritional/dietary consultation and specialized wound care services. As the surveyor is exploring the care processes, he or she also would return to the nursing unit where the patient resides to discuss the findings. It may be that a new theme or area of focus—such as infection control—emerges from this tracer process. The surveyor would then explore this new area more thoroughly and ask other surveyors at your hospital to explore infection control in their tracers to determine if similar findings exist in other tracer patients.

Your organization can help staff learn about this process by conducting your own tracer rounds in conjunction with the PPR and even on a weekly, monthly, or quarterly basis. See page 71 for information on how to perform your own tracer. This exercise could be conducted by a single person or by a team from your organization. For example, the JCAHO coordinator or performance improvement director may perform a mock tracer by selecting a patient and developing sample questions about the care provided to this mock patient. Or your organization may want to enlist the help of various organization leaders and key staff, such as someone involved in medication management or infection control. A team approach allows more staff to get involved in creating sample questions and to bring their unique expertise to their interactions with staff throughout your organization.

In exercises to conduct mock tracers, staff members who are knowledgeable about JCAHO standards can play the role of surveyors and visit the areas your organization has mapped out. The mock surveyors could observe direct care being provided, conduct staff interviews, review records, ask staff about processes and any related performance improvement/measurement issues, and so on to help staff become more comfortable with this process. The tracing of individuals throughout an organization and resulting interaction between surveyors and staff are probably the most dramatic differences that will be apparent to your staff. Helping staff to understand that, for example, surveyors may have asked in the past about a particular policy and will now, instead, be looking at how a process was carried out will be key to a successful survey. The focus is on patients, not on policies. See Sidebar 5-3 to develop sample questions staff can use to prepare for the on-site survey.

Conducting mock tracer activities will allow your leaders and staff to identify performance issues and examine how processes in your organization are linked as a system. This process will, in turn, support your organization's efforts for integrating ongoing standards assessment and compliance in the everyday practices of staff.

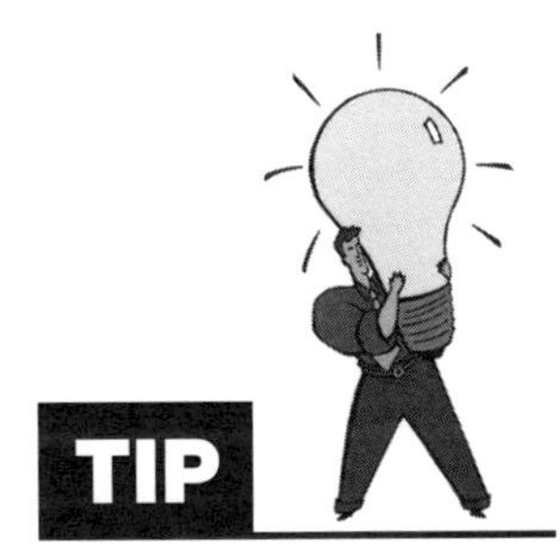

TIP

Conduct a mock tracer for individuals served at your organization so that staff can see how they might be involved in the process. Pull a particular care recipient's record and think of the questions that might arise about how staff met that individual's needs.

For example, if English is a second language for an individual in a tracer, the surveyor may ask how the staff member communicated with that patient, client, or resident to gather information during the assessment process or how education was provided about his or her procedure or care. At that time, the surveyor may ask to see the organization's assessment protocol as well as the human resources file for the staff member involved in the individual's care. By logically working through this process, staff members can get a better feel for how the tracer will work and how their actions make a difference.

Sidebar 5-3: Developing Sample Questions

To involve staff in the survey process, consider asking each department or unit to work with the JCAHO coordinator or quality improvement team to create a list of sample questions that deal with how they deliver safe, high-quality care, treatment, and services. In a long term care organization, staff might decide to create sample survey questions dealing with residents who are receiving rehabilitation therapies. Questions might deal with how staff members are assessing and reassessing the resident's needs, educating the resident and enlisting the resident in creating care plans, and assessing and managing pain. Or home care staff might come up with questions about infection control. These questions might include, What are the most common infections? How do you and your organization work to prevent infections? In addition to helping staff members become more comfortable in thinking about the role that their daily work plays in meeting standards and, therefore, the on-site survey, the thought that goes into creating and answering these questions may spur new quality improvement initiatives in your organization.

System Tracer Activity. In addition to tracing individuals throughout your organization, surveyors will trace specific systems that deal with care. For most organizations, surveyors will address the systems of medication management, infection control, and data use for 2004. Topics of system tracers may change, though, from year to year as the health care environment changes, and, in small organizations, only one system tracer will be used. A system for medication management could involve following the path of a particular medication through selection, procurement, storage, prescribing or ordering, preparing, dispensing, administration, and monitoring for effects. Surveyors will then meet with your organization's staff members to discuss their overall medication management system.

In the medication management system tracer, participants from your organization might include a direct care or service representative from the following areas:

- Clinical staff members who have a role in medication management processes as part of the direct care, treatment, or services they render. These staff members might include nurses, physicians, therapists, dietitians, and others.
- Clinician from the pharmacy or consultant pharmacist who is knowledgeable about the selection of medications available for use and medication monitoring
- Staff responsible for educating both staff and patients, residents, or clients about medication
- Clinical staff who may provide additional perspectives about specific populations of patients, residents, or clients
- Performance improvement staff, if medication management performance improvement initiatives are being conducted or have been conducted. This person may already be slated to participate in the system tracer process as a clinician. For example, a therapist may be on the medication performance improvement team and could fill both of these roles during the on-site survey.
- Laboratory specialist
- Environmental safety personnel, such as pump maintenance

In addition, surveyors will visit areas relevant to medication management processes in your organization and talk with available staff members about their roles in medication management.

For the infection control system tracer, your organization should choose staff members who are able to address issues related to the infection control program in all major departments or areas within your organization. These issues include clinical staff such as physicians, nurses, pharmacists, and laboratorians. Clinicians who are knowledgeable about the selection of medications available for use and for pharmacokinetic monitoring should also participate, as well as clinicians from the laboratory, when applicable, who are knowledgeable about microbiology. Other participants include all clinical staff members specifically involved in infection control, along with a sample of individuals from your organization who are involved in the direct provision of care, treatment, and services. Staff responsible for the physical plant and your organization's leadership will also be involved in this aspect of the on-site survey process.

The data use portion of the system tracer process focuses on your organization's use of data to improve the safety and quality of care. Once again, staff participating in this aspect of the survey should be able to discuss issues about the use of data in all major departments or areas within your organization. This includes clinical staff involved in performance improvement and a sample of individuals involved in the direct provision of care, treatment, and services. Representatives of nursing, the medical staff, and pharmacists also will be an important part of this tracer. In addition, a leadership representative and staff members who are knowledgeable about your organization's use of information systems to collect data, analyze data, and report data will participate.

Performing Your Own Tracers

Tracers can be performed in conjunction with the full PPR and option 1 to help your organization and staff get a more complete picture of performance. Conducting your own tracers is not required but can be beneficial because it can accomplish the following:

- Determine the effectiveness of your process design in the delivery of safe, high-quality care
- Generate staff ideas for process improvements
- Identify areas of noncompliance
- Demonstrate the link between JCAHO standards and issues of care within your organization

You can use the same process surveyors follow to conduct your own tracers. When your organization is given access to the PPR tool, you will also receive a summary of your priority focus areas (PFAs).

Consider adapting the following guidelines to your health care setting and to the types of individuals served:

1. When you receive your PFP Summary Report along with access to the PPR, check the report for your top CSGs and PFAs. These lists represent the populations/services from which you may choose individuals for your tracers and important processes/systems you can address for extra focus. For example, if your organization is a behavioral health care clinic, your top CSGs might be behavioral health, chemical dependency, foster care, and outdoor behavioral health; clients chosen for tracers should come from these groups. Your top four PFAs might be communication, organizational structure, information management, and assessment and care/services; you can look more closely at these areas in your organization for your tracers.

2. Select a sample of open-care recipient records. Base your selections on your CSGs. If your PFP information is not yet available, you can still use the criteria discussed earlier. Try to choose care recipients who have received care in as many areas as possible so you will be able to evaluate organizationwide processes and continuity of care.

3. Plan your tracers. Based on the records, make a list of the disciplines or areas that have been involved with each individual's care or treatment. For each area, make another list of representative personnel you will need to interview and applicable standards you will need to address. For example, you may want to have the staff members who actually provided care/services for a specific care recipient (also identified from the medical record) on hand, although any staff members who perform the same function can be interviewed. Inform participants such as attending physicians, staff nurses, pharmacists, therapists, dietitians, laboratory technicians, and others that they will need to be available.

You will also want to include Accreditiation Participation Requirements (APRs), such as compliance with National Patient Safety Goals, and performance measurement requirements (if applicable).

The tracers will depend on individual standards requirements. Staff interviews will occur in all areas. For example, if you are addressing self-medication education for home health patients, you will need to review your organization's educational materials and talk to patients to evaluate the materials' effectiveness. See Figure 5-1 on page 73 for a sample tracer map.

4. Conduct your tracer. Have staff members who are knowledgeable about JCAHO standards play the role of surveyors and visit the areas you have mapped out on your plan. Have them conduct interviews, review records, and so on.

5. Use your results to identify areas for improvement. Compliance issues found during your tracer can help prioritize improvement efforts. For instance, if you find that reassessments for pain are not being performed on a timely basis within your ambulatory center, you may decide to reallocate resources to provide pain management in-services for staff.

Repeat this process a number of times to identify your organization's strengths as well as trends in compliance issues that may need improvement.

Proficiency Testing Validation and Regulatory Review (Laboratory Only). The Proficiency Testing Validation and Regulatory Review, two sepa-

Figure 5-1: Example Tracer Map

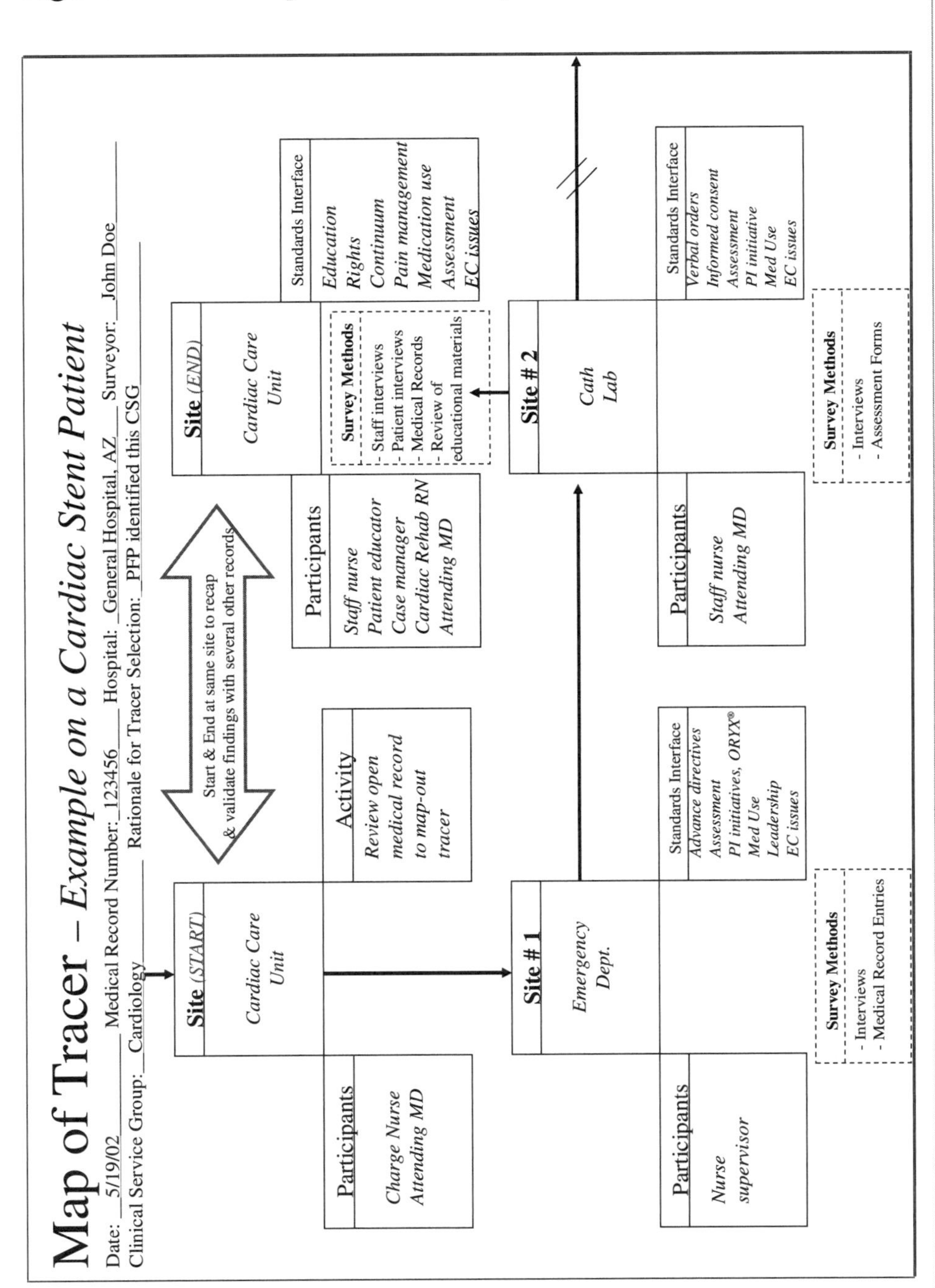

rate sessions, will take place only in a JCAHO laboratory accreditation survey. In Proficiency Testing Validation, surveyors will review the results of proficiency testing and review nonregulated analyte performance criteria if not included in proficiency testing. In the Regulatory Review session, surveyors will verify that your laboratory is performing services according to Centers for Medicare & Medicaid Services (CMS) and state requirements, review Clinical Laboratory Improvement Amendments (CLIA) certificates, validate specialty and subspecialty information, and review state licenses as required of the laboratory and personnel.

Staff who will work with a JCAHO laboratory surveyor as part of this process might include the laboratory administrative director, medical director, and section supervisors.

Special Issue Resolution. This session provides an opportunity for surveyors to follow up on any outstanding issues that could not be resolved in other survey activities. Depending on the findings, this follow-up could involve reviewing policies or procedures, reviewing additional clinical records to follow up on a tracer finding, review of personnel files, or discussions with staff in a specific area. The staff involved in this portion of the on-site survey will vary depending upon the issue.

Daily Briefing. In surveys lasting more than one day, surveyors will summarize for your organization's leadership the activities and findings of a day's survey at a daily briefing. This summary could involve commenting on positive findings or on issues that could lead to compliance problems. Your organization will also have an opportunity to provide any information it did not provide during the previous day. There will be no daily briefing on the last scheduled day of the survey.

Staff involved in daily briefings include your organization's CEO or administrator, along with other senior leaders chosen by your CEO.

Competence Assessment Process. During this session, your staff and surveyors will discuss the overall design of competence assessment processes for staff, licensed independent practitioners (LIPs), and other credentialed practitioners, including the strengths and areas for improvement within that process. Orientation, training, and education for these groups will also be discussed. This session will help surveyors determine your organization's level of compliance with relevant standards. This session is not a record audit.

Staff from your organization selected for participation should include the people responsible for human resources, education, and the assessment of staff competency. Your organization should also expect to have the individuals responsible for assessing LIP and other credentialed practitioner competency available, as well as the human resources manager or other person who has authority to access personnel and credentials files.

Medical Staff Credentialing and Privileging (Hospital Only). In hospital surveys, surveyors will meet with your staff during this session to discuss your facility's process for collecting relevant data for appointment decisions. Other items for discussion include the following:

- Consistent implementation of the credentialing and privileging process for the medical staff and other LIPs who are privileged through the medical staff process
- Processes for granting privileges and for appropriate delineation of privileges
- Practitioners practicing within the limited scope of delineated privileges
- Links between the results of peer review and focused monitoring to the credentialing and privileging process
- Identification of vulnerabilities in the credentialing, privileging, and appointment process

Your organization's medical staff president, medical director, and medical staff coordinator, along with representatives from the medical staff credentials committee, should be prepared to participate in this discussion.

Environment of Care Session. The Environment of Care (EC) session will be divided into two parts. Group discussion on managing risk in your organization's environment will make up 30% of the session, with surveyor observation and evaluation of your organization's performance in managing EC risk comprising the remaining 70%. First, surveyors will review your organization's annual evaluations of your EC risk management plan and team meeting minutes of the EC multidisciplinary team to become better acquainted with your environment. Then, surveyors and staff will discuss the environment to identify strengths and vulnerabilities in your organization's environment and actions necessary to address any vulnerabilities and assess your organization's compliance with relevant standards. Surveyors will then identify the EC management process they would like to observe based on the prior discussion. The surveyor will trace the EC activity throughout your organization to see it in action and to identify any risk points in the process. Surveyors may also review EC issues as they move through your organization during a tracer.

Staff from your organization who participate in the EC review process should be able to address issues in all major departments or areas. For example, the person or persons designated by your organization's leadership to coordinate safety management activities and security management activities will play a major role in this part of the on-site survey. Other staff who will be involved include the person who manages your organization's facilities, handles emergency management activities, and manages building utility systems. The person responsible for maintaining medical and laboratory equipment will also participate, except in behavior health care organizations. The leader of the EC team or safety committee and your organization's leaders should round out the group of participants. At complex organizations that have decentralized EC management activities at remote sites, staff members responsible for managing these activities should be available either in person or by conference call to talk with JCAHO surveyors.

***Life Safety Code*® Building Tour.** Surveyors will tour those buildings of your organization that are required to be designed and maintained according to *Life Safety Code*® *(LSC)* requirements. Through this tour, surveyors will identify any vulnerabilities in your organization's process for designing and maintaining buildings according to the code and for identifying and resolving code issues. Surveyors will then determine your organization's level of compliance with *LSC* requirements.

The person who manages your organization's facility will meet with a JCAHO surveyor for the *LSC* tour, along with any other relevant staff that your organization wishes to include.

Leadership Session. During the leadership activity, your organization's leadership will meet with surveyors to discuss specific survey issues. That discussion could include your organization's performance in PFAs and the surveyors' assessment of links between standards compliance and PFA issues. The goal of this session is to "connect the dots" and to tie specific findings to broader issues that affect your organization. Performance in systems of care, standards, or Accreditation Participation Requirements, including JCAHO's National Patient Safety Goals, might also be discussed.

As expected, a variety of your organization's leaders play a role in this session. This session includes at least one member of the governing body or a trustee. If you are a single-owner organization, this individual may also be the CEO. Senior leaders from all programs and services also will be involved, although the individuals and titles may vary depending on the type of organization being surveyed. Examples of senior leaders include CEO, COO, CFO, CIO, administrator, laboratory medical director, vice president for clinical services, nurse executive, and director of patient services or branch manager. Elected and appointed leaders of the medical staff, if applicable to your organization, will also participate.

CEO Exit Briefing and Organization Exit Conference. At the end of the survey, your organization's CEO will meet with surveyors to discuss the outcome of the survey, present and explain the Accreditation Report, and discuss any concerns with the report. Surveyors will also identify any special arrangements for the Organization Exit Conference. For example, your CEO may not, at that time, wish to share the Accreditation Report with other representatives of your organization, or perhaps your CEO would like the accreditation results to be shared verbally. During the Exit Conference, your CEO and any other organization leaders invited by him or her will hear from surveyors about standards compliance issues.

Your organization's CEO should attend this final session of the on-site survey. Your CEO may also wish to invite other senior leaders and staff to attend. This decision is left to your CEO.

Interaction with Surveyors

The goal is not for physicians or any other staff to memorize the standards. Standards have been developed, with significant input from physicians and other health care providers, as a format or structure that can be used to guide operational activities in a health care organization. If physicians and the HCO staff look at the standards as best practices that will promote high-quality patient care, they will find that compliance is a by-product. See Sidebar 5-4 below for more information on physician involvement in the survey.

Sidebar 5-4: Engaging Physicians in the Survey Process

Following are suggestions an organization can use to encourage its medical staff to participate in the survey process (while this information focuses specifically on physicians, consider adapting these ideas for other staff):

- Medical staff should be encouraged to interact with JCAHO surveyors. Surveyors will not expect a regurgitation of JCAHO standards and the hospital's mission. Instead, they will want to discuss systems and processes—already an area which physicians are very familiar with.
- A physician's main objective is to provide high-quality, safe patient care. The new survey process plays to that strength. Physicians can help the surveyors to understand the process within the health care organization.
- Surveyors will also try to learn more about physician priorities and plans to improve care.
- Under the new survey process, surveyors are likely to monitor a patient's entire episode of care from a patient's first entry into the hospital, to the operating room, to the postanesthesia care unit, to the intensive care unit, to the medical surgical unit, and on to discharge
- Surveyors will look for care provided to patients, so it is important to fully understand the care physicians provide as the patient transitions through the care delivery process*

JCAHO has also announced that surveyors will specifically seek physician input when the hospital completes the Periodic Performance Review (PPR), develops plans of action, and participates in evaluation sessions.

---

* Sentana Bayside Hospital: Sentana Bayside 2004 JCAHO Medical Staff Educational Manual. Virginia Beach, Virginia, 2004.

CHAPTER SIX

EVIDENCE OF STANDARDS COMPLIANCE AND MEASURES OF SUCCESS

As part of Shared Visions–New Pathways®, your organization must either document how it has come into compliance with any standards identified as not compliant during the survey or state why your organization believes it was in compliance with the standards at the time of survey. This report, known as the Evidence of Standards Compliance (ESC), is a natural extension of the new accreditation philosophy that encourages continuous standards compliance.

An Overview of ESC and MOS

Before JCAHO surveyors leave your organization, they will share with your CEO a report of their findings. The survey findings also will be posted on your organization's password-protected extranet site, provided there are no flagged items or adverse decisions, approximately 48 hours after the conclusion of the on-site evaluation.

An ESC is required for all EPs that are included in the Requirements for Improvement section of the Accreditation Decision Report. Your organization can submit one of two types of ESC to show that the standard has been brought into compliance. Both types of ESC, which must address compliance at the EP level, are equally important and equally correct in demonstrating standards compliance. In addition, your ESC report can contain both types of ESCs, which are described below:

A *corrective ESC* details the corrective actions you have taken to come into compliance with a standard and should include, if applicable, a measure of success (MOS). An MOS is a numerical or quantifiable measure that demonstrates if an action has been effective and is also being sustained. This process simply asks your organization to detail the actions taken—not just planned—

to come into compliance with a standard and to identify the MOS that will be used to assure sustained compliance.

A *clarifying ESC* demonstrates why you believe your organization was actually in compliance with a standard scored not compliant during survey. You do not need to submit an MOS for this type of ESC. If your organization chooses to submit clarifying ESCs, you will need to review a larger sample size than the one used during the on-site evaluation and convey that information to JCAHO. If there is not adequate evidence to support your organization's clarification submission, your organization will be required to demonstrate compliance with the standard by submitting a second ESC. In this case, the organizations will still need to submit correct ESC within the original time frame of 90 days after survey.

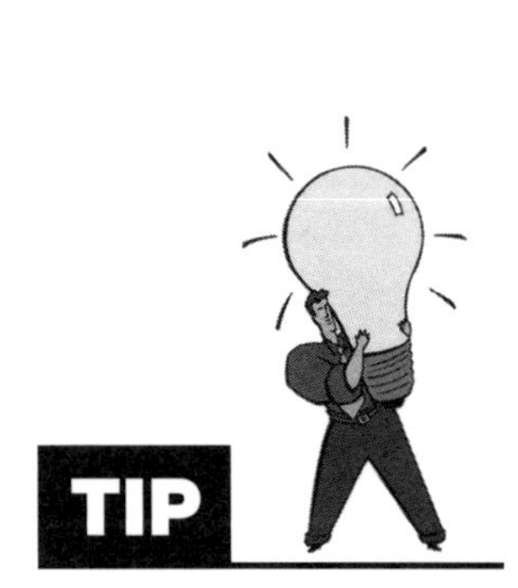

Provide some type of oversight for the ESC process, perhaps an administrator, quality improvement staff member, or your organization's performance improvement steering committee. Allow for any necessary education of these "assessors" on the ESC process and then ask them to work with staff to carry out your organization's compliance plans. Finally, determine a communication process—written, verbal, or electronic—to report progress to staff and leaders as appropriate.

Until July 2005, your organization will have 90 days after your survey to come into compliance with any issues identified during the on-site evaluation. The 90-day time frame recognizes that organizations surveyed during this period will not have had the benefit of submitting and completing the Periodic Performance Review (PPR) to help identify areas of noncompliance. Organizations surveyed beginning in July 2005 will be the first to have submitted their PPR at the midpoint of their accreditation cycle, so after that time it is anticipated that your organization will have 45 days to submit an ESC. Your organization's prior accreditation decision will remain in effect during this submission time.

JCAHO Central Office staff will evaluate your organization's ESC by using the scoring guidelines. These guidelines will be familiar to your organization because they are the same set of rules used by surveyors during the on-site evaluation and used by you to conduct the full PPR or PPR option 1. These universal and objective guidelines also eliminate the need to engage in an appeal's process following your survey. To have the ESC successfully accepted, your organization must demonstrate that you have resolved all requirements for improvement. Your organization should expect a final decision letter shortly after the ESC has been rendered.

If your first ESC is found to be acceptable, your decision will be "Accredited," and you will submit the data for any required MOS for each EP four months later. An unacceptable ESC will trigger a "Provisional Accreditation" decision and require your organization to submit an acceptable ESC within 30 days. If the second ESC is accepted, your organization's accreditation decision will remain "Provisional Accreditation" until acceptable results of the corresponding MOS are submitted four months later. A second ESC found to be unacceptable will prompt a recommendation for "Conditional Accreditation" to JCAHO's Accreditation Committee.

JCAHO Central Office staff also will review MOS results, when required. If the MOS results are found to be acceptable, your organization will not need to take any further action. If your organization had received "Provisional Accreditation," the decision also will change to "Accredited." An "Accredited" organization that submits unacceptable MOS will have its status changed to "Provisional

Accreditation," and a second set of MOS must be submitted in another four months. An organization that receives "Provisional Accreditation" because of an unacceptable ESC submission and submits unacceptable MOS will have a "Conditional Accreditation" recommendation presented to JCAHO's Accreditation Committee.

If a second MOS submission is found to be acceptable, the decision will be changed to "Accredited," and no further action is required. A second unacceptable MOS will bring a "Conditional Accreditation" recommendation before the Accreditation Committee.

Educating Staff and Determining Staff Involved

In most organizations, your JCAHO coordinator and performance improvement team or director will play the lead roles in the ESC process. The ESC will also require teamwork across the organization and depend upon the specific EP found out of compliance.

If your organization is found out of compliance with any EPs, you will have to move quickly to address the issues. The knowledge gained by your staff during the PPR process will help you complete the ESC process, as will the additional educational information for staff and the suggested actions in this chapter.

First, immediately following the on-site survey, your JCAHO coordinator, CEO, and other managers will want to review the final report and give special attention to any requirements for improvement. Listing the relevant standards and EPs for distribution to staff will also be helpful. Members of your organization's planning team, along with those involved in the review of the final report, can then work together to develop strategy. Consider the following questions:

- What standards are identified as "not compliant?"
- What are the related EPs scored partial or insufficient compliance?
- What action is necessary to come into compliance with the requirement for improvement?
- Who are the staff members responsible for the action?
- What is the MOS?
- What is the time frame?

Once those questions have been answered, small team meetings also may be used to bring the ESC issues to the department or unit level. Staff members at this level will need to know exactly what they need to do to help your organization demonstrate compliance. In-service training sessions may help to educate staff about how to comply with related policies or procedures. Brainstorming sessions also may be helpful, in addition to asking staff members in the specific areas how they would go about complying with standards and demonstrating that compliance as part of their daily routines. In some organizations, compliance may turn out to be a matter of better documenting actions.

If your organization is submitting MOS, staff will need to understand that submitting MOS is essentially a way of using data to "prove" that you are doing what you say you will. Staff members should recognize that their actions are important in creating MOS and that the data gathering process may include staff interviews. Other sources in the MOS data gathering process might include building inspection, performance improvement data, staff testing after in-services, general observations, and record reviews. While your organization is not required to address supplemental recommendations as part of the ESC, it is a good idea to include them in your plan to reach 100% compliance 100% of the time. Supplemental findings will be entered into the Priority Focus Process for your organization's next survey.

To help your organization focus ESC education efforts, consider the following example. An organization that was found to be out of compliance with standards requiring ongoing collection of surveillance data on nosocomial infections may use the brief space provided on the ESC section of the extranet to explain the following corrective action:

Director of Nursing and Infection Control Coordinator reeducated on policy of daily collection of nosocomial infection data. Daily collection of data will occur at the start of their shift. New nosocomial infection data collection tool developed and implemented. Daily updates given to patient (or client or resident) department heads regarding this unit's nosocomial infection rates.

The evaluation method may be presented, for example, as follows:

Weekly audit of infection data collection tool to determine if daily collection of surveillance data on nosocomial infections is ongoing.

The MOS would be entered as "100%."

An organization submitting a clarifying ESC for this issue might provide, for example, the following explanation:

Collection of surveillance data on nosocomial infections has been occurring daily. Data collection tools are stored in a binder in the Infection Control Coordinator's office. Binders were available to the surveyors for review. Internal audit of binder revealed that daily collection of nosocomial infections has occurred 96% of the time over the previous two years.

Regardless of whether your organization has to complete the ESC process, the weeks and months following the departure of the on-site survey team offer additional opportunities to educate staff about how they fit into your institution's accreditation goals. Explaining the meaning of your organization's accreditation decision will help staff members see how their work contributed to the process. In addition, the accreditation decision offers an opportunity to emphasize that continuous improvement of performance is an institutional goal and the JCAHO report supports that goal by highlighting areas in which improvement is the highest priority.

Your organization's CEO and JCAHO coordinator can accomplish these goals in a variety of ways. An organizationwide celebration may be in order, or an all-staff memo or voice mail may be used to share information about your accreditation decision. See Sidebar 6-1 on page 84 for a sample staff memo. Your organization can then provide additional information through memos, internal newsletters, e-mails, and bulletin boards.

This information might, for example, explain that your organization has now completed its first full experience with the Shared Visions–New Pathways initiative. Staff should know that the new accreditation decision process, which your organization completed, is different in the following ways:

- It reflects a focus on ongoing standards compliance
- It is more credible, assuring the public that your organization has demonstrated full compliance with rigorous, national standards
- It is based on the number of standards that are scored not compliant
- It focuses less on scores and more on using the standards to achieve and maintain excellent operational systems in which your staff play an integral role

If your organization has emphasized an accreditation score in the past, you may want to let staff know that there is no overall score or grid element score with the new accreditation decision process. However, the accreditation report does list requirements for improvement by PFA (processes, systems, or structures important to providing safe, quality care in a health care organization).

To help staff understand the distinctions among accreditation decisions, you may choose to share with them not only the definition of the decision your organization receives but also the definitions of all the decisions possible.

The accreditation decision category definitions are as follows:

***Accredited*—**An organization demonstrates compliance with all of the standards at the time of the on-site survey or resolves requirements for improvement via an acceptable ESC submission.

***Provisional Accreditation*—**Not all requirements for improvement have been addressed in the ESC submission, or the organization has failed to achieve an appropriate level of sustained compliance as determined by an MOS result

***Conditional Accreditation*—**Number of standards scored not compliant is between two and three standard deviations above the mean number of not compliant standards for organizations in that accreditation program. The organization must undergo an on-site follow-up survey.

***Preliminary Denial of Accreditation*—**Number of standards scored not compliant is three or more standard deviations above the mean number of not compliant standards for organizations in that accreditation program. There is justification to deny accreditation, but the decision is subject to appeal.

***Denial of Accreditation*—**The organization has been denied accreditation, and all review and appeal opportunities have been exhausted.

***Preliminary Accreditation*—**The organization demonstrates compliance with selected standards in the first of two surveys conducted under the Early Survey Policy Option 1. This decision remains in effect until one of the other official accreditation decision categories is assigned, based on a complete survey against all applicable standards approximately six months later.

Sidebar 6-1: Sample Memo to Staff Regarding Accreditation Decision

This sample letter may be helpful in communicating information about your organization's accreditation to staff. The memo provides an opportunity to inform staff about the work that went into achieving accreditation, the importance of accreditation to your organization, and any follow-up activities that will be required.

Dear Staff:

I am pleased to inform you that we have received accreditation from the Joint Commission on Accreditation of Healthcare Organizations (JCAHO). Congratulations!

You should be proud that our focus on the most challenging goal—to continuously raise quality and safety to higher levels—has resulted in this national recognition. Accreditation is proof of our organizationwide commitment to provide quality care on an ongoing basis.

Your teamwork and dedication made this possible. I thank you for your efforts and encourage you to remain committed to ongoing compliance with JCAHO standards. Together with your input, we will be able to continue to provide positive outcomes for our patients.

I should also note that our JCAHO surveyors identified several areas of standards compliance that must be addressed in the near future. These areas offer improvement opportunities, and our success in resolving these issues will be dependent upon your ideas and assistance. Specific information will be communicated in coming days.

Again, congratulations on a job well done!

Sincerely,

CEO/Administrator

CHAPTER SEVEN

INTRACYCLE SURVEY EVENTS

Random unannounced surveys, unannounced surveys, and extension surveys remain a part of the accreditation process, although the Shared Visions–New Pathways® initiative will bring a number of changes to these familiar on-site evaluations. Changes to the on-site survey, including use of the Priority Focus Process (PFP) and tracer activities, which will affect intracycle survey events have already been discussed in previous chapters in this book. This chapter provides an explanation of intracycle survey events.

An Overview of Random Unannounced Surveys

JCAHO conducts random unannounced surveys in a 5% random sample of accredited organizations to determine ongoing compliance with standards. Your organization is eligible to receive a random unannounced survey 9 to 30 months following your full triennial survey. You will receive no notice for this type of survey. Organizations that volunteer during 2004 and 2005 to participate in pilot testing of the unannounced triennial survey process will not be in the pool for random unannounced surveys.

If your organization is selected for a random unannounced survey, the scope and focus of this evaluation is based on both fixed and variable components. Variable components are identified through the PFP, in which presurvey information is processed to indicate specific priority focus areas (PFAs) to be evaluated during these surveys. The presurvey information may include previous survey findings; data from your organization's application for accreditation; data from JCAHO's Quality Monitoring System, including sentinel events and complaints; ORYX® core measure data; and external data (for example, from state and federal agencies).

Fixed components are based on the three most serious PFAs for a given year and the National Patient Safety Goals as they apply to the services provided by

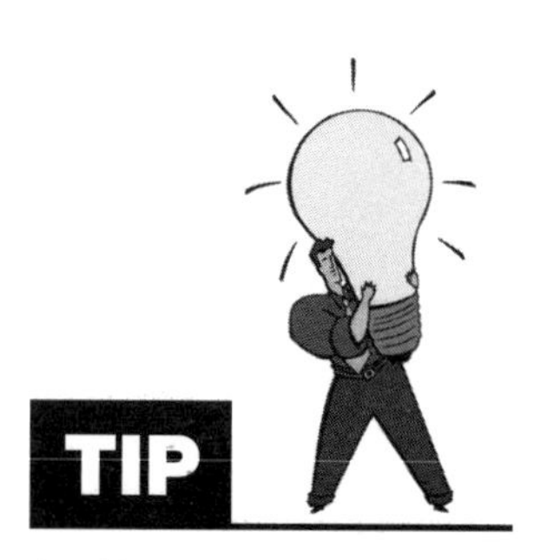

Consider creating a telephone hotline for staff members to call if they have pressing questions that require an immediate answer or if they believe there is a serious issue related to safe, quality care. Depending on your organization, the performance improvement manager or JCAHO coordinator may be the best person to handle these calls. Or perhaps the risk manager or another respected leader who cuts across disciplines could be designated for this responsibility.

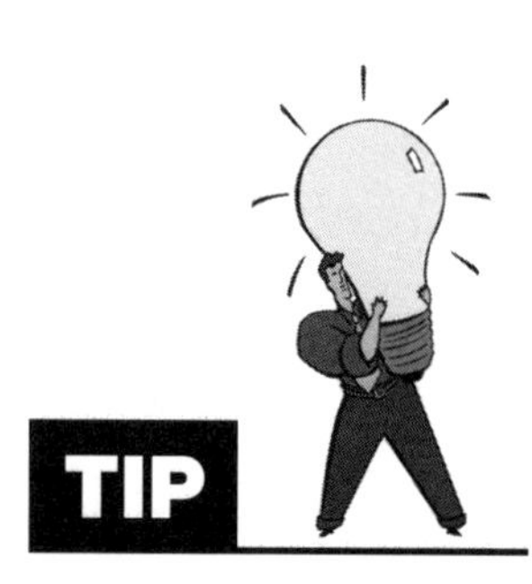

Check out the newsletter *Joint Commission Perspectives®* for a list of PFAs and National Patient Safety Goals that will guide random unannounced surveys in 2005.

your organization. The three PFAs applicable, for example, to random unannounced surveys in 2004 are staffing, infection control, and medication management. Both the applicable PFAs and the National Patient Safety Goals are updated each year.

The review of variable components takes precedence over the review of fixed components, so information will be accessed immediately before a random unannounced survey to make sure that it is up-to-date. The surveyor will review all variable components identified for your organization and then address fixed components as time allows.

Staff Education and Determining Staff Involved

Because your organization is striving for 100% compliance with standards 100% of the time, the random unannounced survey process does not require additional preparations or education beyond the strategies you already have in place. Your organization should continue emphasizing a commitment to "living" the standards on a daily basis as staff deliver care, treatment, and services and use the random unannounced survey as a tool to encourage staff to adopt this philosophy. A brief discussion about random unannounced surveys might, for example, be included in your organization's general efforts to educate staff about JCAHO accreditation. All organization staff should also be aware that the results of a random unannounced survey might generate follow-up activities and can affect your organization's accreditation decision. This knowledge may, in turn, prompt staff to speak up when they see an issue as part of their work or to bring ideas for improvement opportunities to your organization's performance improvement director. Supervisors and staff should be aware that their efforts to continuously comply with relevant standards and National Patient Safety Goals could be tested at any time.

If your organization is selected for a random unannounced survey, the on-site visit typically takes only one day and is conducted by one surveyor. The surveyor will seek out your CEO or the individual in charge of your organization, begin the opening conference, then move on to other activities. The staff involved will depend upon your organization but will likely include representatives from each major department or unit. For details of which staff members are involved in which aspects of the survey process, please refer to Chapter 5.

An Overview of Extension Surveys

An extension survey may be conducted at an accredited organization or a site that is owned and operated by an accredited organization. This type of survey is performed if your organization's accreditation will not expire for at least nine months and at least one of the following conditions applies:

- You have begun offering a new service or program for which JCAHO has standards
- Your organization has changed ownership, and there have been signifi-

cant changes in your management and clinical staff or operating policies and procedures
- You have begun offering at least 25% of your services in a new location or in a physical plant that has been significantly altered
- Your organization's capacity to provide services has expanded by 25% or more (calculated by patient, resident, or client volume, pieces of equipment, or other relevant measures)
- You have begun providing a more intensive level of service
- Your organization has merged/consolidated with or acquired an unaccredited site, service, or program for which JCAHO has standards
- Your organization has merged/consolidated with or acquired another accredited organization whose accreditation is due to expire within three months of the merger/consolidation or acquisition

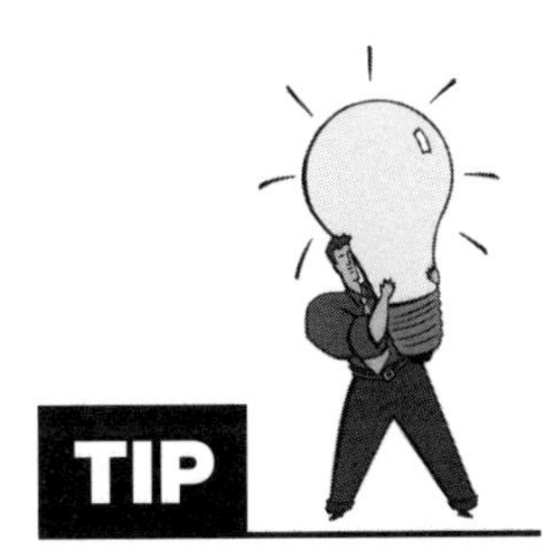

An accreditation fair may help keep staff focused on your organization's commitment to patient safety and quality improvement and offer educational opportunities in a fun atmosphere. Your organization could solicit staff to volunteer to plan the fair. Think of a theme and fun activities that can be used to teach staff what they need to know to consistently deliver safe, high-quality care.

An extension survey may also be conducted if, due to unusual or compelling reasons, you have requested that your current accreditation be extended beyond the conclusion of your accreditation cycle. The length of the survey will be from one to five days. The surveyor will use the same type of approach in an extension survey as a full survey. Because of the varying circumstance for scheduling extension surveys, there may be considerable variation in the specific issues addressed by the surveyor. The extension survey is not a full survey.

Staff Participation in an Extension Survey and Determining Staff Involved

An extension survey will require some staff participation. To prepare, your organization will want to inform all staff about the extension survey, perhaps in the form of a memo from your CEO, and discuss the upcoming extension survey at all staff meetings. The changes in your organization that prompted the need for the extension survey will help guide specific education efforts. For example, if your organization has merged or acquired another organization, it will be important to assess how the two organizations have educated staff about important aspects of care that can be impacted by a merger or acquisition. From there, you can begin to coordinate policies and procedures and assess standards compliance to determine which areas may require additional or concentrated staff education.

By knowing what to expect and what is expected of them, staff members in your organization can perform to the best of their ability for care recipients. Specific topics to address in education efforts might include the following:

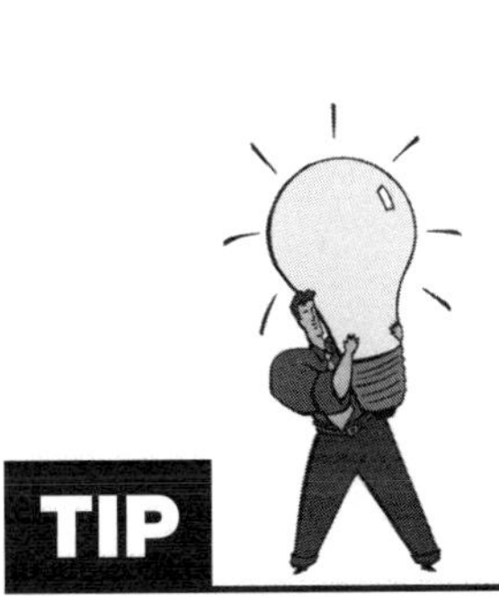

Contact your JCAHO Account Representative to find out if your organization qualifies for an extension survey and how to go about requesting an extension survey. The main JCAHO telephone number for questions about accreditation, scheduling, agendas, process, and so forth is 630/792-3007.

- The reason for the extension survey
- How quality can be impacted by the recent change that necessitated the extension survey
- Specific areas that have been impacted by the recent change, and how standards can provide assistance in provision of quality care in these areas

- How compliance will be assessed
- How to access information needed to identify opportunities for improvement and to develop plans of action

To accomplish this process, your organization's leaders and staff will want to work together closely. Expanding the performance improvement team to include representatives from the new service or organization/site that triggered the need for an extension survey is critical to success.

An Overview of For-Cause Surveys

For-cause surveys are conducted when JCAHO becomes aware of potentially serious care-and-safety or standards compliance issues. The reasons for conducting a for-cause survey include any event or series of events in an organization that raises concerns about the following:

- A continuing threat to patient care or safety
- Serious and/or multiple significant deficiencies in standards compliance
- Credible allegations that an organization has falsified accreditation information

Types of serious events or concerns that may trigger a for-cause survey include allegations of fraud; deaths, including suicide and treatment mishaps such as medication errors; or physical environmental and safety concerns, including fire deaths, murders, and other safety-related fatalities. For-cause surveys can be classified either as unannounced or unscheduled.

For-cause unannounced surveys are conducted without any advance notice and can include all of an organization's services or only those areas where a serious concern may exist. This type of survey typically takes one or two days, depending on the seriousness of the for-cause event, and may occur at any point in the accreditation cycle.

Organizations that receive a for-cause unscheduled survey are given 24 to 48 hours' notice of the site visit before it is conducted. Unscheduled surveys are conducted instead of unannounced surveys if no substantive corrective action is feasible within the 24- to 48-hour time frame and if the issue under investigation does not involve an allegation of falsifying information.

Results from either type of for-cause survey may require follow-up activities, such as providing Evidence of Standards Compliance, and may affect your organization's existing accreditation decision. Organizations that refuse to allow JCAHO to conduct an unannounced survey may face having their decision changed to "Denial of Accreditation."

If your organization does undergo a for-cause survey, leaders and the JCAHO accreditation coordinator should expect to be involved in the on-site process and any required follow-up activities.

APPENDIX A

CYCLE-CHART OF THE ACCREDITATION PROCESS

Use the cycle-charts of the accreditation process in this appendix to help educate staff where each step in the process occurs in relation to the other steps in the continuum that leads to accreditation. Each page highlights one activity and a general description of that activity appears in the center. The time frame for each activity is also provided. Look to your program-specific accreditation manual for a more robust description of each activity and which activities apply to your program.

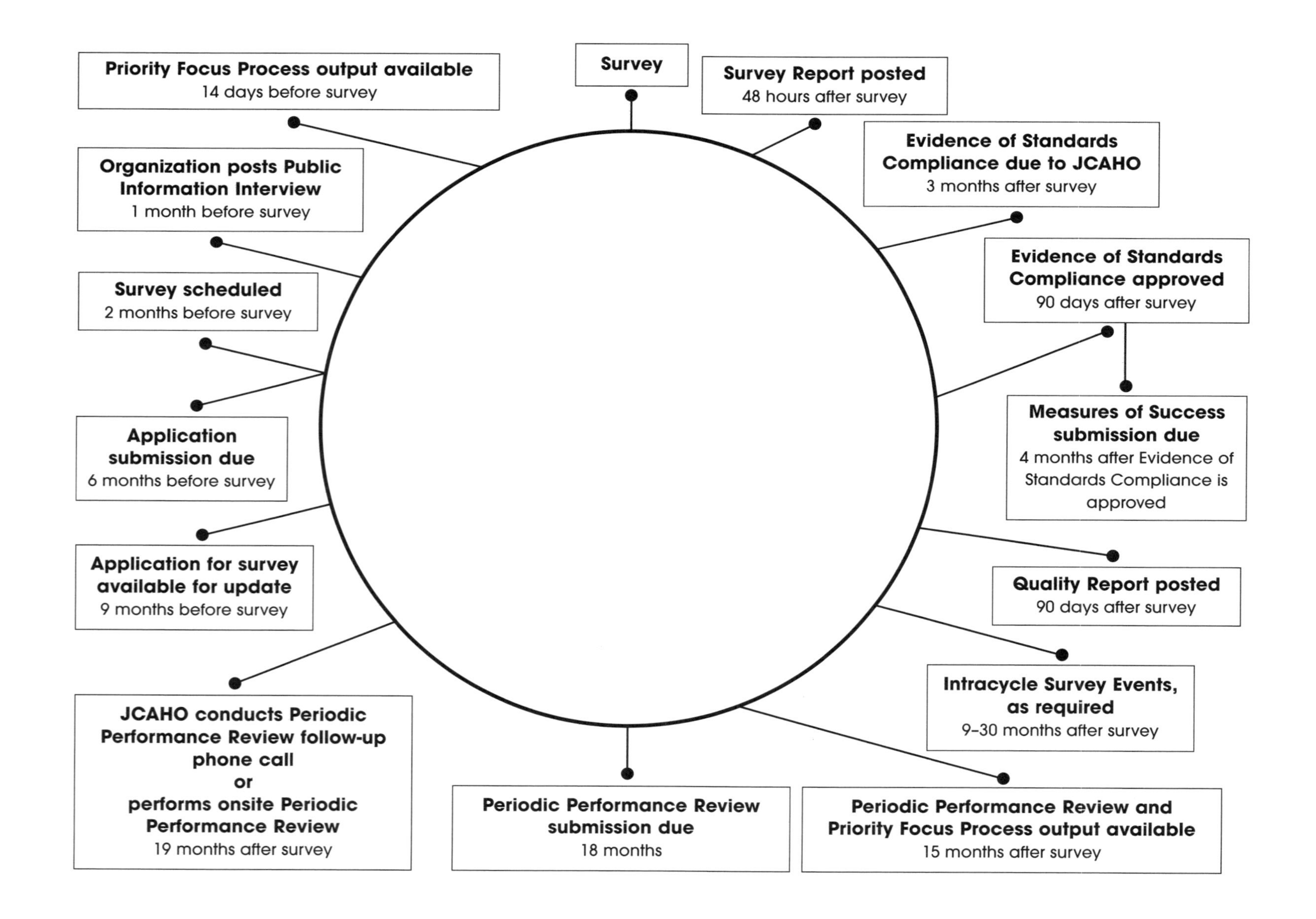

Priority Focus Process output available
14 days before survey
Survey
Survey Report posted
48 hours after survey
Evidence of Standards Compliance due to JCAHO
3 months after survey
Evidence of Standards Compliance approved
90 days after survey
Measures of Success submission due
4 months after Evidence of Standards Compliance is approved
Quality Report posted
90 days after survey
Intracycle Survey Events, as required
9–30 months after survey
Periodic Performance Review and Priority Focus Process output available
15 months after survey
Periodic Performance Review submission due
18 months
JCAHO conducts Periodic Performance Review follow-up phone call
or
performs onsite Periodic Performance Review
19 months after survey
Application for survey available for update
9 months before survey
Application submission due
6 months before survey
Survey scheduled
2 months before survey
Organization posts Public Information Interview
1 month before survey

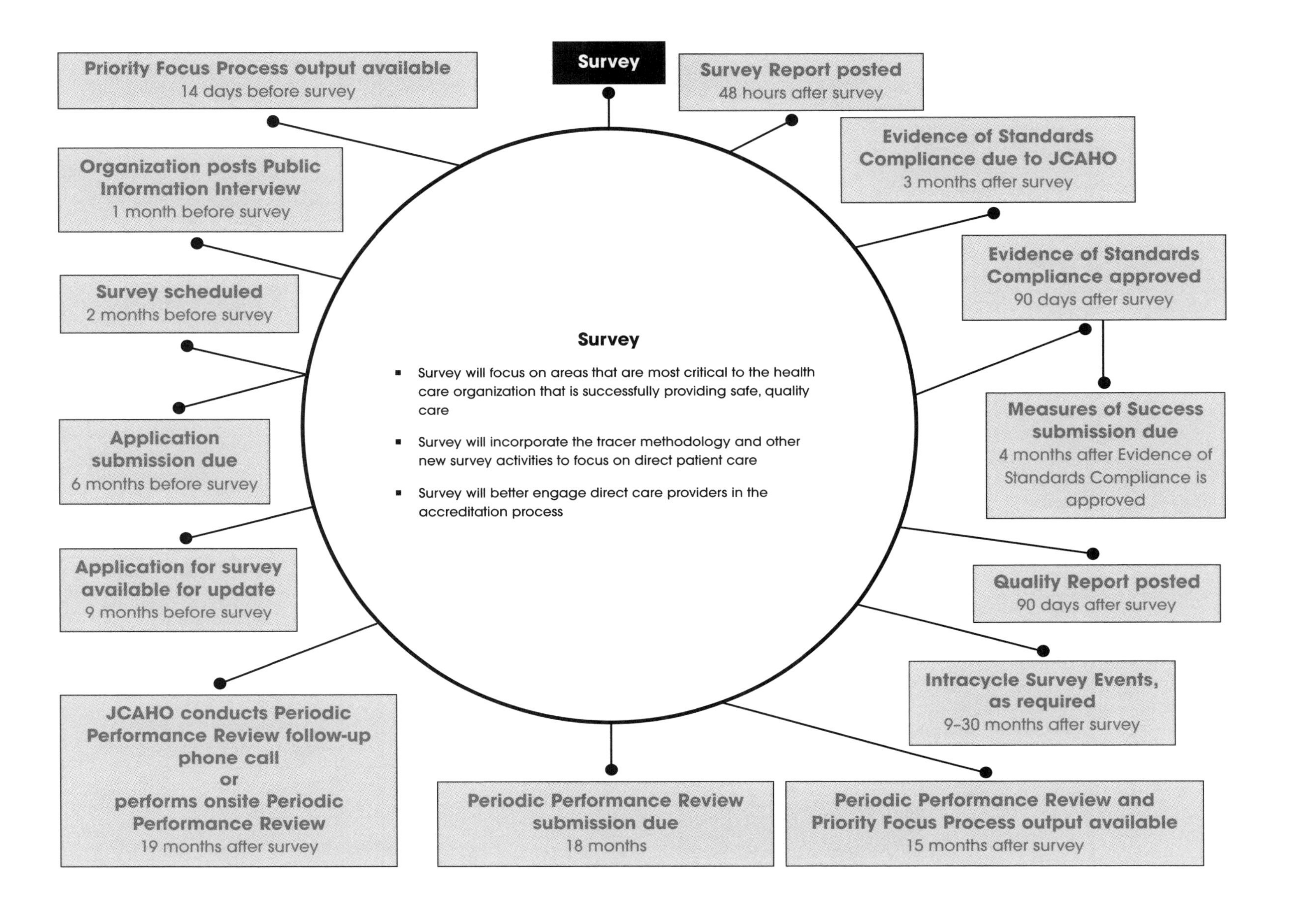
Survey
Survey Report posted
48 hours after survey
Evidence of Standards Compliance due to JCAHO
3 months after survey
Evidence of Standards Compliance approved
90 days after survey
Measures of Success submission due
4 months after Evidence of Standards Compliance is approved
Quality Report posted
90 days after survey
Intracycle Survey Events, as required
9–30 months after survey
Periodic Performance Review and Priority Focus Process output available
15 months after survey
Periodic Performance Review submission due
18 months
JCAHO conducts Periodic Performance Review follow-up phone call
or
performs onsite Periodic Performance Review
19 months after survey
Application for survey available for update
9 months before survey
Application submission due
6 months before survey
Survey scheduled
2 months before survey
Organization posts Public Information Interview
1 month before survey
Priority Focus Process output available
14 days before survey
Survey
Survey will focus on areas that are most critical to the health care organization that is successfully providing safe, quality care
Survey will incorporate the tracer methodology and other new survey activities to focus on direct patient care
Survey will better engage direct care providers in the accreditation process

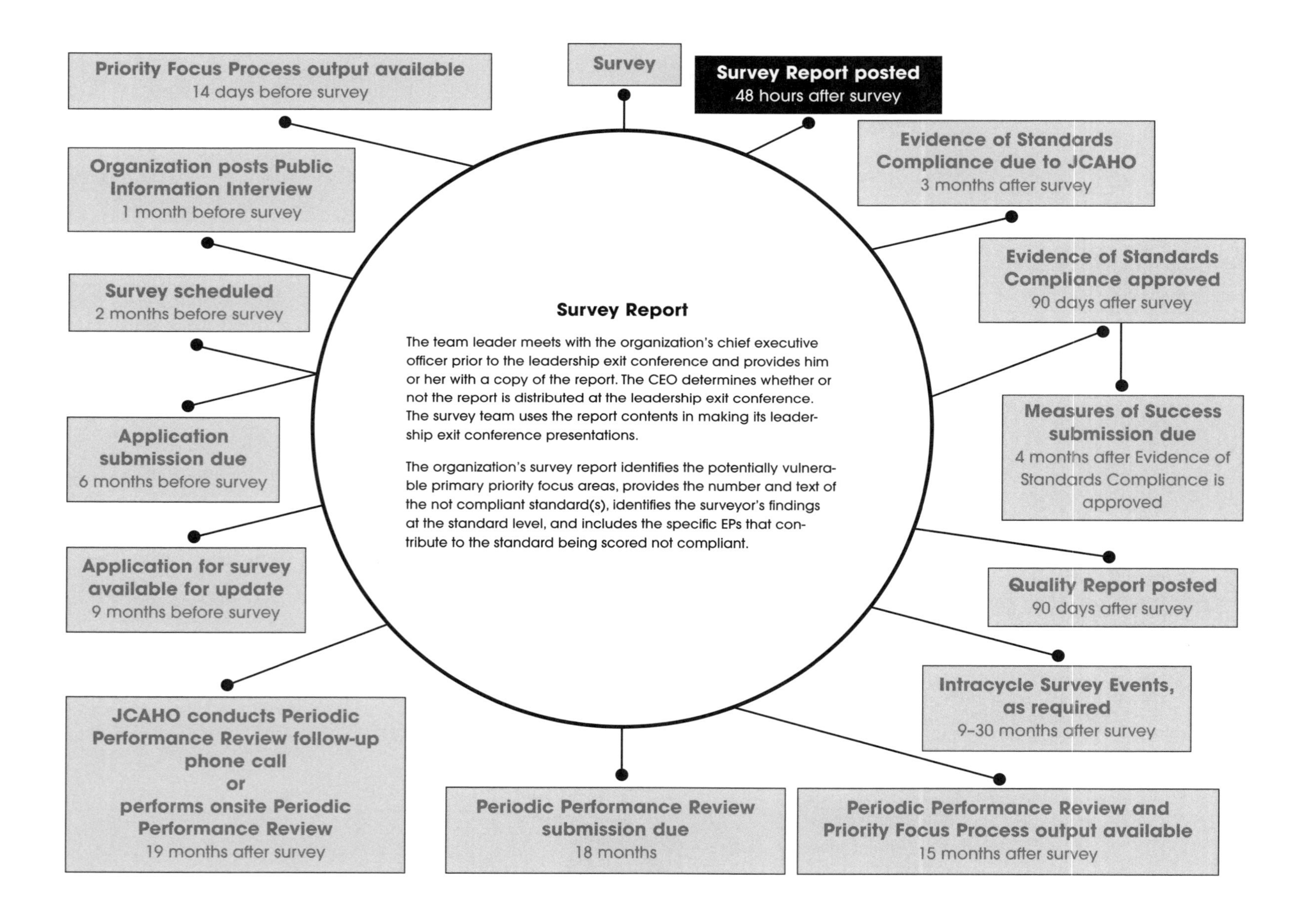
Priority Focus Process output available
14 days before survey
Survey
Survey Report posted
48 hours after survey
Organization posts Public Information Interview
1 month before survey
Evidence of Standards Compliance due to JCAHO
3 months after survey
Survey scheduled
2 months before survey
Evidence of Standards Compliance approved
90 days after survey
Survey Report
The team leader meets with the organization's chief executive officer prior to the leadership exit conference and provides him or her with a copy of the report. The CEO determines whether or not the report is distributed at the leadership exit conference. The survey team uses the report contents in making its leadership exit conference presentations.
The organization's survey report identifies the potentially vulnerable primary priority focus areas, provides the number and text of the not compliant standard(s), identifies the surveyor's findings at the standard level, and includes the specific EPs that contribute to the standard being scored not compliant.
Application submission due
6 months before survey
Measures of Success submission due
4 months after Evidence of Standards Compliance is approved
Application for survey available for update
9 months before survey
Quality Report posted
90 days after survey
Intracycle Survey Events, as required
9–30 months after survey
JCAHO conducts Periodic Performance Review follow-up phone call
or
performs onsite Periodic Performance Review
19 months after survey
Periodic Performance Review submission due
18 months
Periodic Performance Review and Priority Focus Process output available
15 months after survey

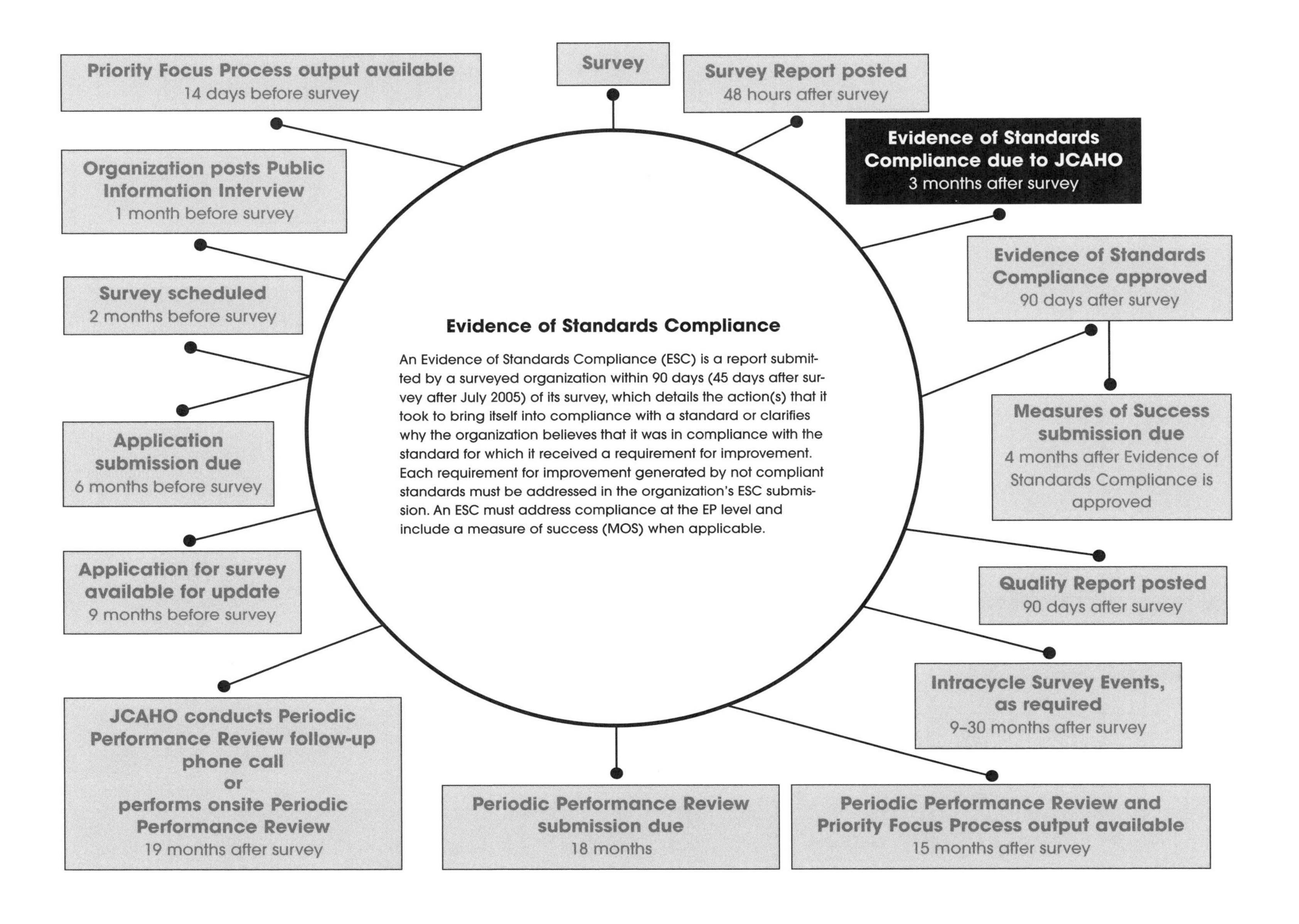
Survey
Survey Report posted
48 hours after survey
Evidence of Standards Compliance due to JCAHO
3 months after survey
Evidence of Standards Compliance approved
90 days after survey
Measures of Success submission due
4 months after Evidence of Standards Compliance is approved
Quality Report posted
90 days after survey
Intracycle Survey Events, as required
9–30 months after survey
Periodic Performance Review and Priority Focus Process output available
15 months after survey
Periodic Performance Review submission due
18 months
JCAHO conducts Periodic Performance Review follow-up phone call
or
performs onsite Periodic Performance Review
19 months after survey
Application for survey available for update
9 months before survey
Application submission due
6 months before survey
Survey scheduled
2 months before survey
Organization posts Public Information Interview
1 month before survey
Priority Focus Process output available
14 days before survey
Evidence of Standards Compliance
An Evidence of Standards Compliance (ESC) is a report submitted by a surveyed organization within 90 days (45 days after survey after July 2005) of its survey, which details the action(s) that it took to bring itself into compliance with a standard or clarifies why the organization believes that it was in compliance with the standard for which it received a requirement for improvement. Each requirement for improvement generated by not compliant standards must be addressed in the organization's ESC submission. An ESC must address compliance at the EP level and include a measure of success (MOS) when applicable.

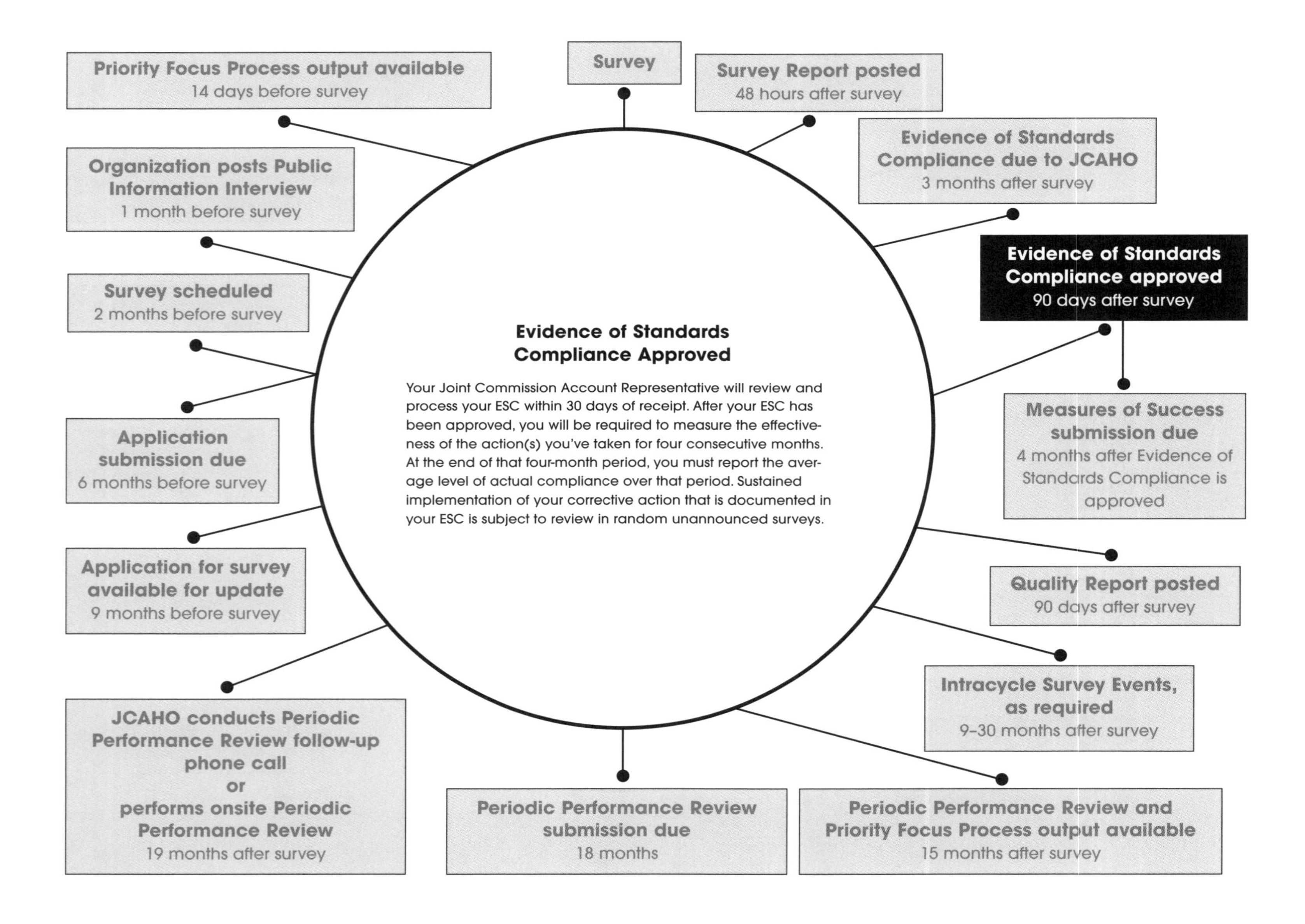
Priority Focus Process output available
14 days before survey
Survey
Survey Report posted
48 hours after survey
Organization posts Public Information Interview
1 month before survey
Evidence of Standards Compliance due to JCAHO
3 months after survey
Survey scheduled
2 months before survey
Evidence of Standards Compliance approved
90 days after survey
Evidence of Standards Compliance Approved
Your Joint Commission Account Representative will review and process your ESC within 30 days of receipt. After your ESC has been approved, you will be required to measure the effectiveness of the action(s) you've taken for four consecutive months. At the end of that four-month period, you must report the average level of actual compliance over that period. Sustained implementation of your corrective action that is documented in your ESC is subject to review in random unannounced surveys.
Application submission due
6 months before survey
Measures of Success submission due
4 months after Evidence of Standards Compliance is approved
Application for survey available for update
9 months before survey
Quality Report posted
90 days after survey
Intracycle Survey Events, as required
9–30 months after survey
JCAHO conducts Periodic Performance Review follow-up phone call
or
performs onsite Periodic Performance Review
19 months after survey
Periodic Performance Review submission due
18 months
Periodic Performance Review and Priority Focus Process output available
15 months after survey

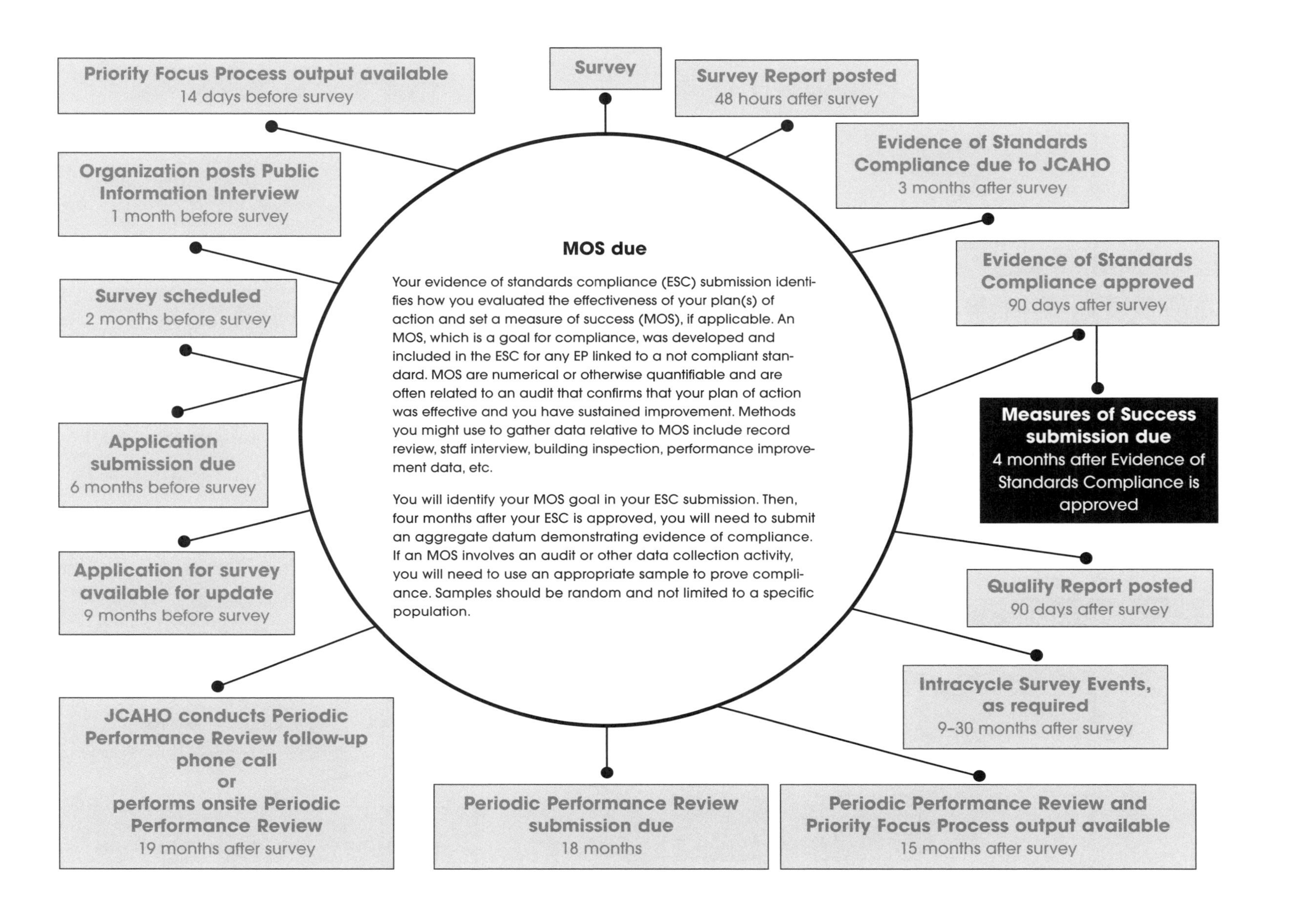
Priority Focus Process output available
14 days before survey
Survey
Survey Report posted
48 hours after survey
Evidence of Standards Compliance due to JCAHO
3 months after survey
Evidence of Standards Compliance approved
90 days after survey
Measures of Success submission due
4 months after Evidence of Standards Compliance is approved
Quality Report posted
90 days after survey
Intracycle Survey Events, as required
9–30 months after survey
Periodic Performance Review and Priority Focus Process output available
15 months after survey
Periodic Performance Review submission due
18 months
JCAHO conducts Periodic Performance Review follow-up phone call
or
performs onsite Periodic Performance Review
19 months after survey
Application for survey available for update
9 months before survey
Application submission due
6 months before survey
Survey scheduled
2 months before survey
Organization posts Public Information Interview
1 month before survey
MOS due
Your evidence of standards compliance (ESC) submission identifies how you evaluated the effectiveness of your plan(s) of action and set a measure of success (MOS), if applicable. An MOS, which is a goal for compliance, was developed and included in the ESC for any EP linked to a not compliant standard. MOS are numerical or otherwise quantifiable and are often related to an audit that confirms that your plan of action was effective and you have sustained improvement. Methods you might use to gather data relative to MOS include record review, staff interview, building inspection, performance improvement data, etc.
You will identify your MOS goal in your ESC submission. Then, four months after your ESC is approved, you will need to submit an aggregate datum demonstrating evidence of compliance. If an MOS involves an audit or other data collection activity, you will need to use an appropriate sample to prove compliance. Samples should be random and not limited to a specific population.

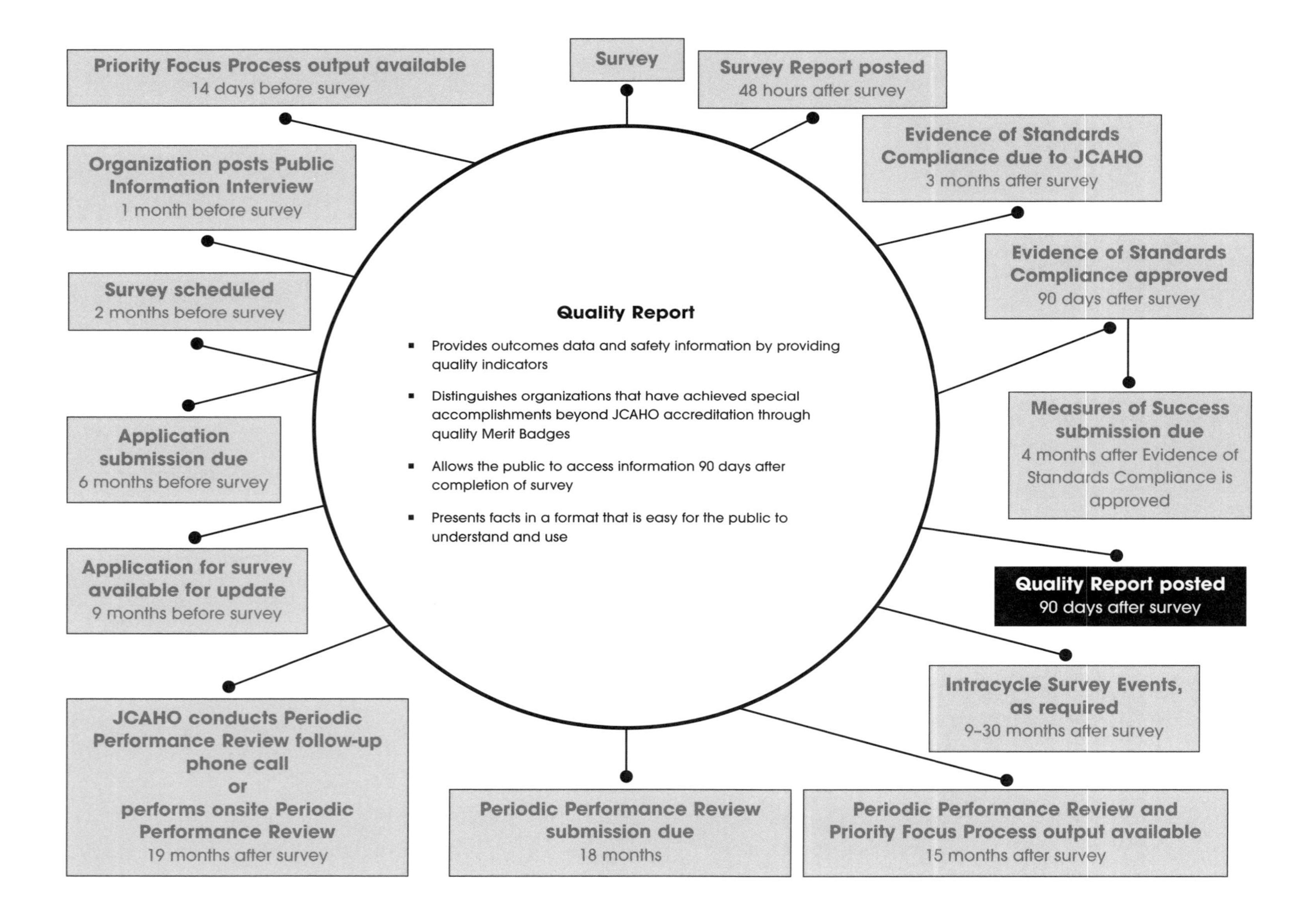
Priority Focus Process output available
14 days before survey
Organization posts Public Information Interview
1 month before survey
Survey scheduled
2 months before survey
Application submission due
6 months before survey
Application for survey available for update
9 months before survey
JCAHO conducts Periodic Performance Review follow-up phone call
or
performs onsite Periodic Performance Review
19 months after survey
Survey
Survey Report posted
48 hours after survey
Evidence of Standards Compliance due to JCAHO
3 months after survey
Evidence of Standards Compliance approved
90 days after survey
Measures of Success submission due
4 months after Evidence of Standards Compliance is approved
Quality Report posted
90 days after survey
Intracycle Survey Events, as required
9–30 months after survey
Periodic Performance Review and Priority Focus Process output available
15 months after survey
Periodic Performance Review submission due
18 months
Quality Report
Provides outcomes data and safety information by providing quality indicators
Distinguishes organizations that have achieved special accomplishments beyond JCAHO accreditation through quality Merit Badges
Allows the public to access information 90 days after completion of survey
Presents facts in a format that is easy for the public to understand and use

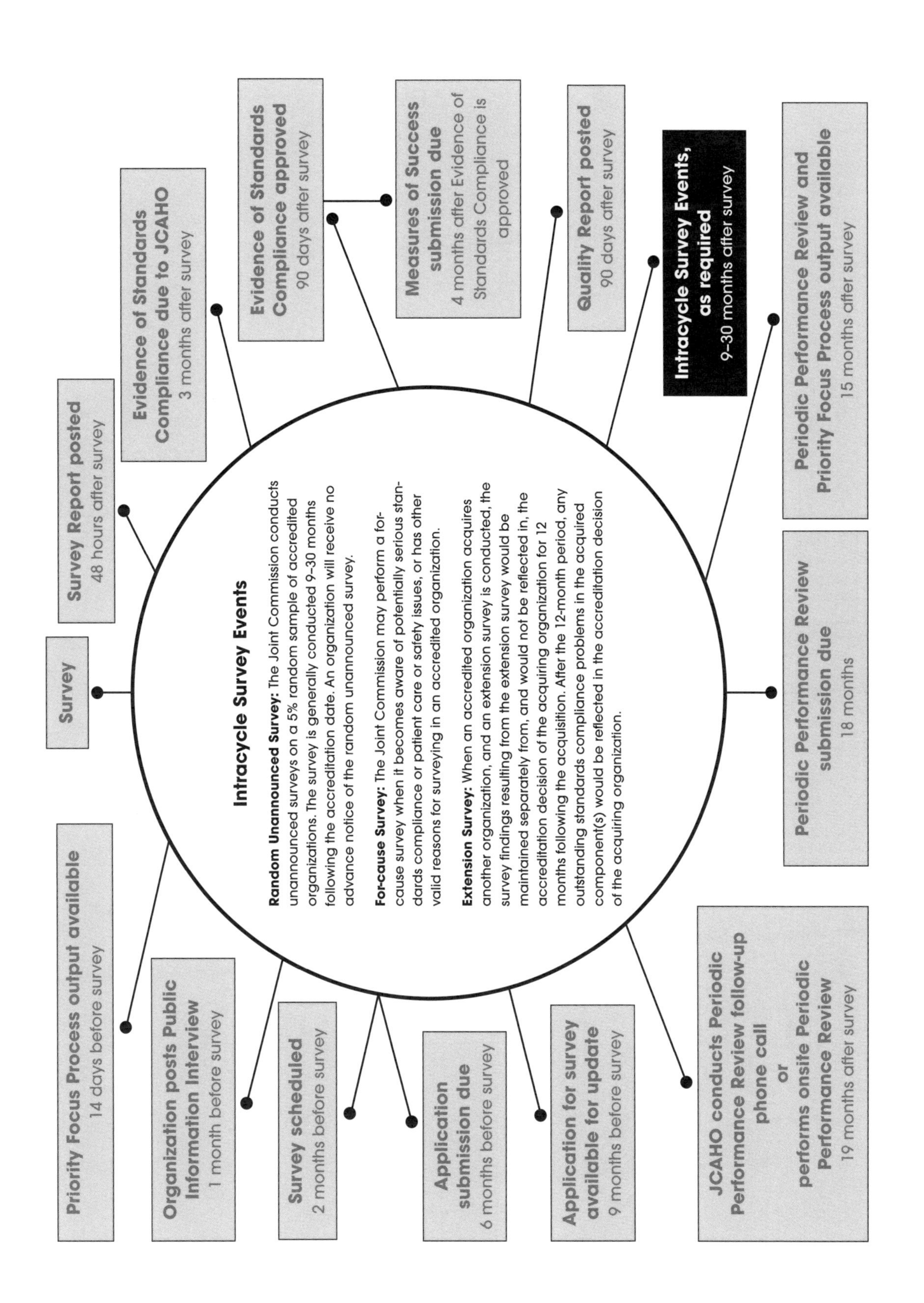
Intracycle Survey Events
Random Unannounced Survey: The Joint Commission conducts unannounced surveys on a 5% random sample of accredited organizations. The survey is generally conducted 9–30 months following the accreditation date. An organization will receive no advance notice of the random unannounced survey.
For-cause Survey: The Joint Commission may perform a for-cause survey when it becomes aware of potentially serious standards compliance or patient care or safety issues, or has other valid reasons for surveying in an accredited organization.
Extension Survey: When an accredited organization acquires another organization, and an extension survey is conducted, the survey findings resulting from the extension survey would be maintained separately from, and would not be reflected in, the accreditation decision of the acquiring organization for 12 months following the acquisition. After the 12-month period, any outstanding standards compliance problems in the acquired component(s) would be reflected in the accreditation decision of the acquiring organization.
Survey
Survey Report posted
48 hours after survey
Evidence of Standards Compliance due to JCAHO
3 months after survey
Evidence of Standards Compliance approved
90 days after survey
Measures of Success submission due
4 months after Evidence of Standards Compliance is approved
Quality Report posted
90 days after survey
Intracycle Survey Events, as required
9–30 months after survey
Periodic Performance Review and Priority Focus Process output available
15 months after survey
Periodic Performance Review submission due
18 months
JCAHO conducts Periodic Performance Review follow-up phone call
or
performs onsite Periodic Performance Review
19 months after survey
Application for survey available for update
9 months before survey
Application submission due
6 months before survey
Survey scheduled
2 months before survey
Organization posts Public Information Interview
1 month before survey
Priority Focus Process output available
14 days before survey

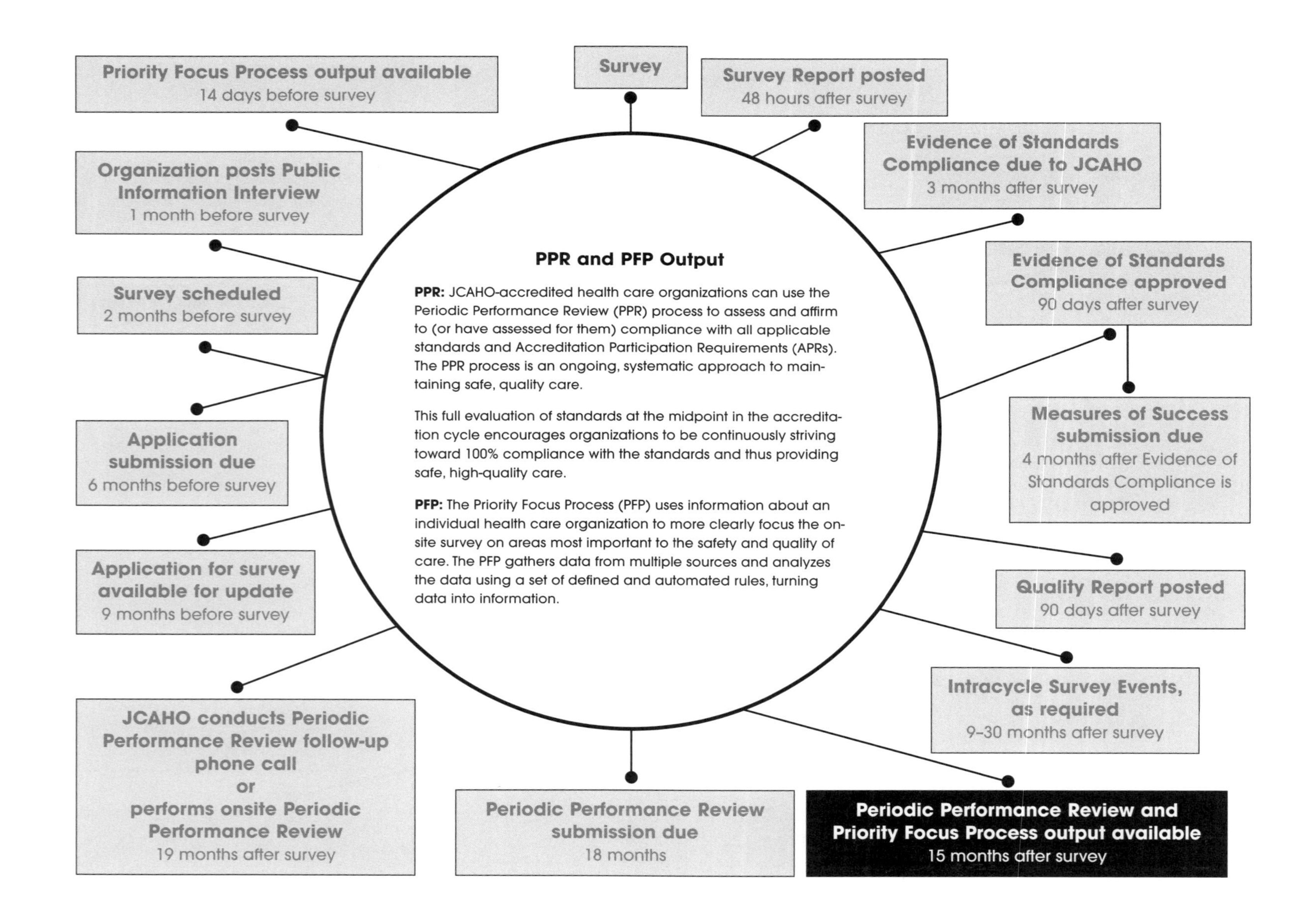

PPR and PFP Output

PPR: JCAHO-accredited health care organizations can use the Periodic Performance Review (PPR) process to assess and affirm to (or have assessed for them) compliance with all applicable standards and Accreditation Participation Requirements (APRs). The PPR process is an ongoing, systematic approach to maintaining safe, quality care.

This full evaluation of standards at the midpoint in the accreditation cycle encourages organizations to be continuously striving toward 100% compliance with the standards and thus providing safe, high-quality care.

PFP: The Priority Focus Process (PFP) uses information about an individual health care organization to more clearly focus the on-site survey on areas most important to the safety and quality of care. The PFP gathers data from multiple sources and analyzes the data using a set of defined and automated rules, turning data into information.

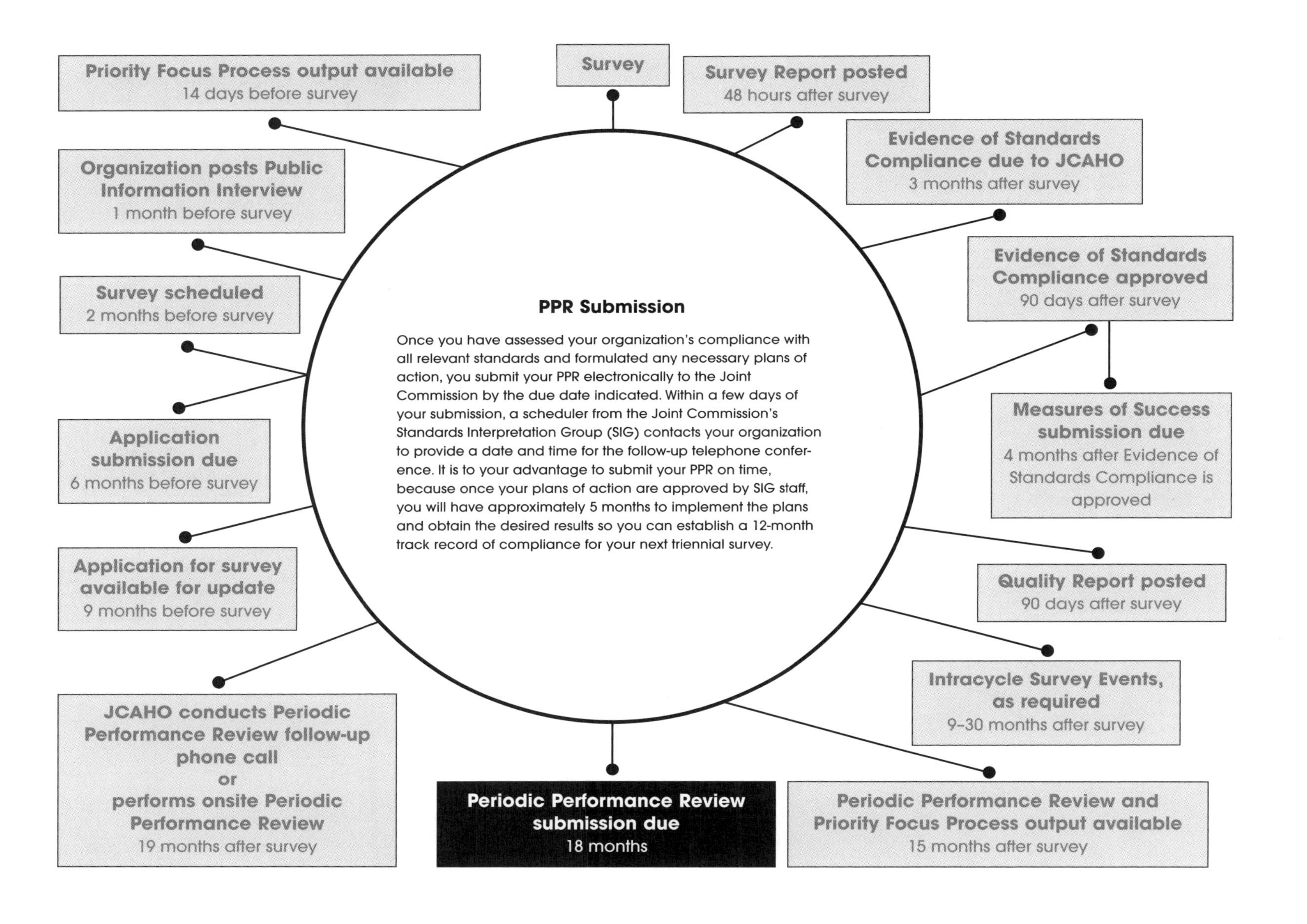
Survey
Survey Report posted
48 hours after survey
Evidence of Standards Compliance due to JCAHO
3 months after survey
Evidence of Standards Compliance approved
90 days after survey
Measures of Success submission due
4 months after Evidence of Standards Compliance is approved
Quality Report posted
90 days after survey
Intracycle Survey Events, as required
9–30 months after survey
Periodic Performance Review and Priority Focus Process output available
15 months after survey
Periodic Performance Review submission due
18 months
JCAHO conducts Periodic Performance Review follow-up phone call
or
performs onsite Periodic Performance Review
19 months after survey
Application for survey available for update
9 months before survey
Application submission due
6 months before survey
Survey scheduled
2 months before survey
Organization posts Public Information Interview
1 month before survey
Priority Focus Process output available
14 days before survey
PPR Submission
Once you have assessed your organization's compliance with all relevant standards and formulated any necessary plans of action, you submit your PPR electronically to the Joint Commission by the due date indicated. Within a few days of your submission, a scheduler from the Joint Commission's Standards Interpretation Group (SIG) contacts your organization to provide a date and time for the follow-up telephone conference. It is to your advantage to submit your PPR on time, because once your plans of action are approved by SIG staff, you will have approximately 5 months to implement the plans and obtain the desired results so you can establish a 12-month track record of compliance for your next triennial survey.

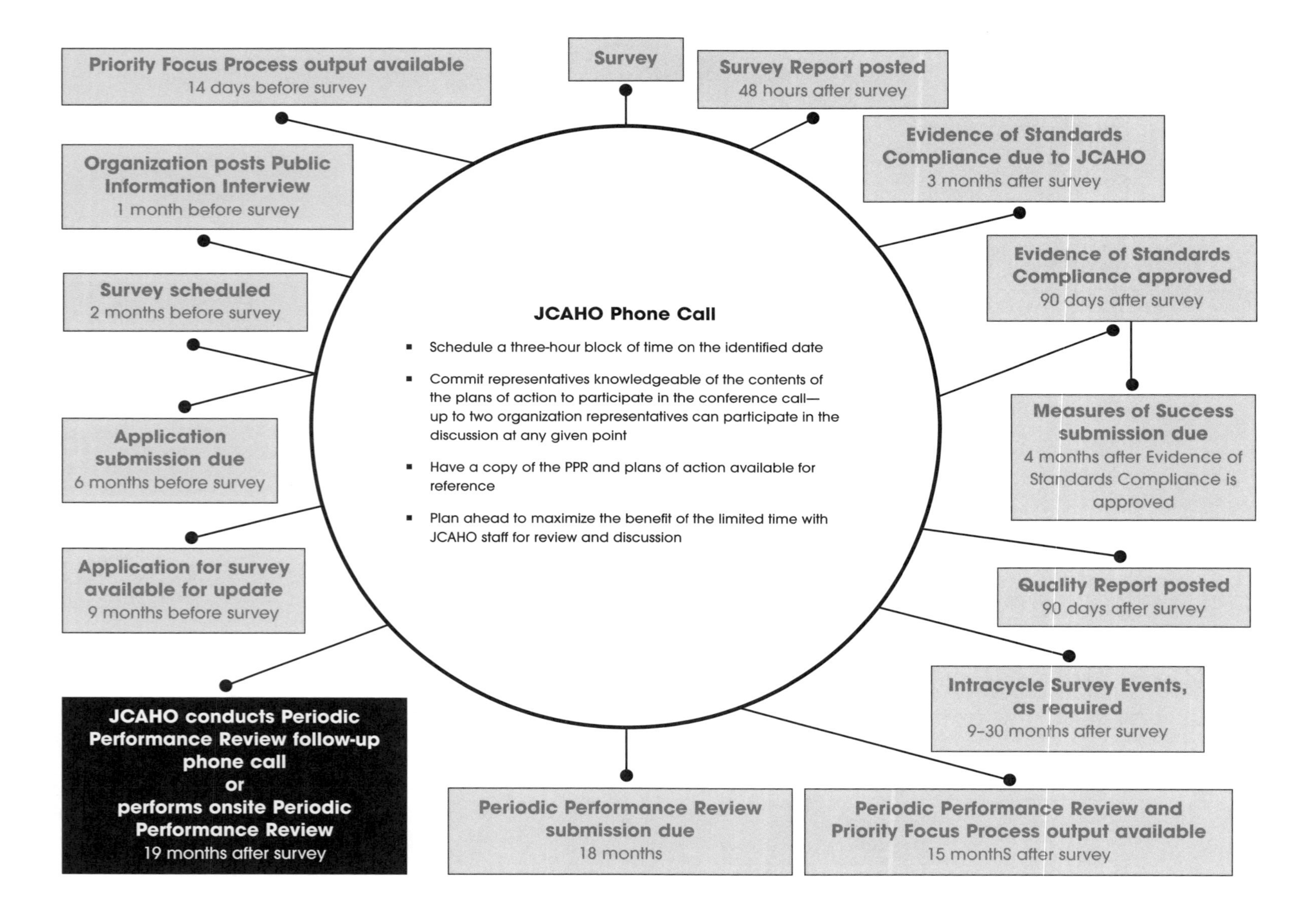
Priority Focus Process output available
14 days before survey
Survey
Survey Report posted
48 hours after survey
Organization posts Public Information Interview
1 month before survey
Evidence of Standards Compliance due to JCAHO
3 months after survey
Survey scheduled
2 months before survey
Evidence of Standards Compliance approved
90 days after survey
JCAHO Phone Call
Schedule a three-hour block of time on the identified date
Commit representatives knowledgeable of the contents of the plans of action to participate in the conference call—up to two organization representatives can participate in the discussion at any given point
Have a copy of the PPR and plans of action available for reference
Plan ahead to maximize the benefit of the limited time with JCAHO staff for review and discussion
Application submission due
6 months before survey
Measures of Success submission due
4 months after Evidence of Standards Compliance is approved
Application for survey available for update
9 months before survey
Quality Report posted
90 days after survey
Intracycle Survey Events, as required
9–30 months after survey
JCAHO conducts Periodic Performance Review follow-up phone call
or
performs onsite Periodic Performance Review
19 months after survey
Periodic Performance Review submission due
18 months
Periodic Performance Review and Priority Focus Process output available
15 monthS after survey

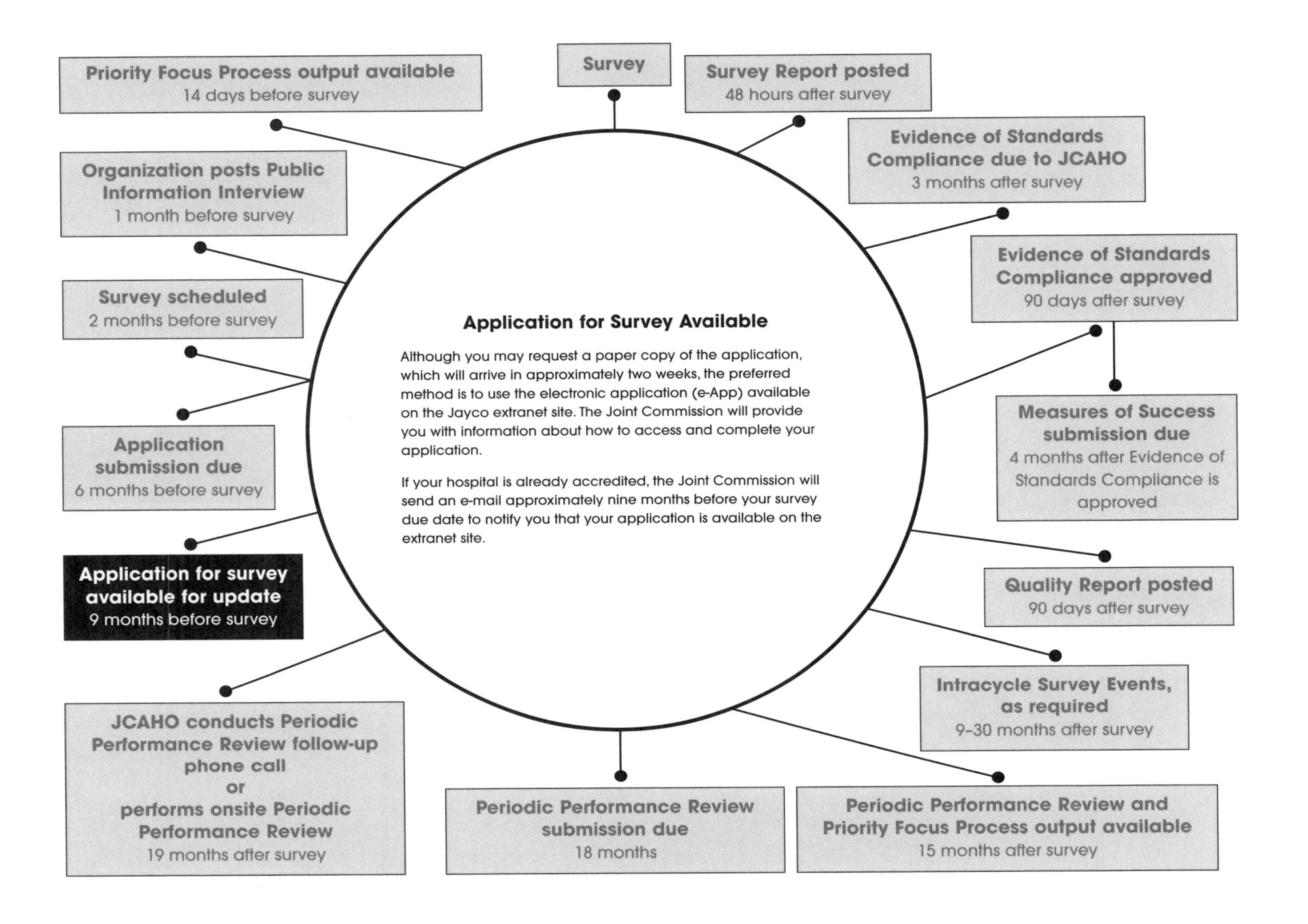
Application for Survey Available
Although you may request a paper copy of the application, which will arrive in approximately two weeks, the preferred method is to use the electronic application (e-App) available on the Jayco extranet site. The Joint Commission will provide you with information about how to access and complete your application.
If your hospital is already accredited, the Joint Commission will send an e-mail approximately nine months before your survey due date to notify you that your application is available on the extranet site.
Application for survey available for update
9 months before survey
Application submission due
6 months before survey
Survey scheduled
2 months before survey
Organization posts Public Information Interview
1 month before survey
Priority Focus Process output available
14 days before survey
Survey
Survey Report posted
48 hours after survey
Evidence of Standards Compliance due to JCAHO
3 months after survey
Evidence of Standards Compliance approved
90 days after survey
Measures of Success submission due
4 months after Evidence of Standards Compliance is approved
Quality Report posted
90 days after survey
Intracycle Survey Events, as required
9–30 months after survey
Periodic Performance Review and Priority Focus Process output available
15 months after survey
Periodic Performance Review submission due
18 months
JCAHO conducts Periodic Performance Review follow-up phone call
or
performs onsite Periodic Performance Review
19 months after survey

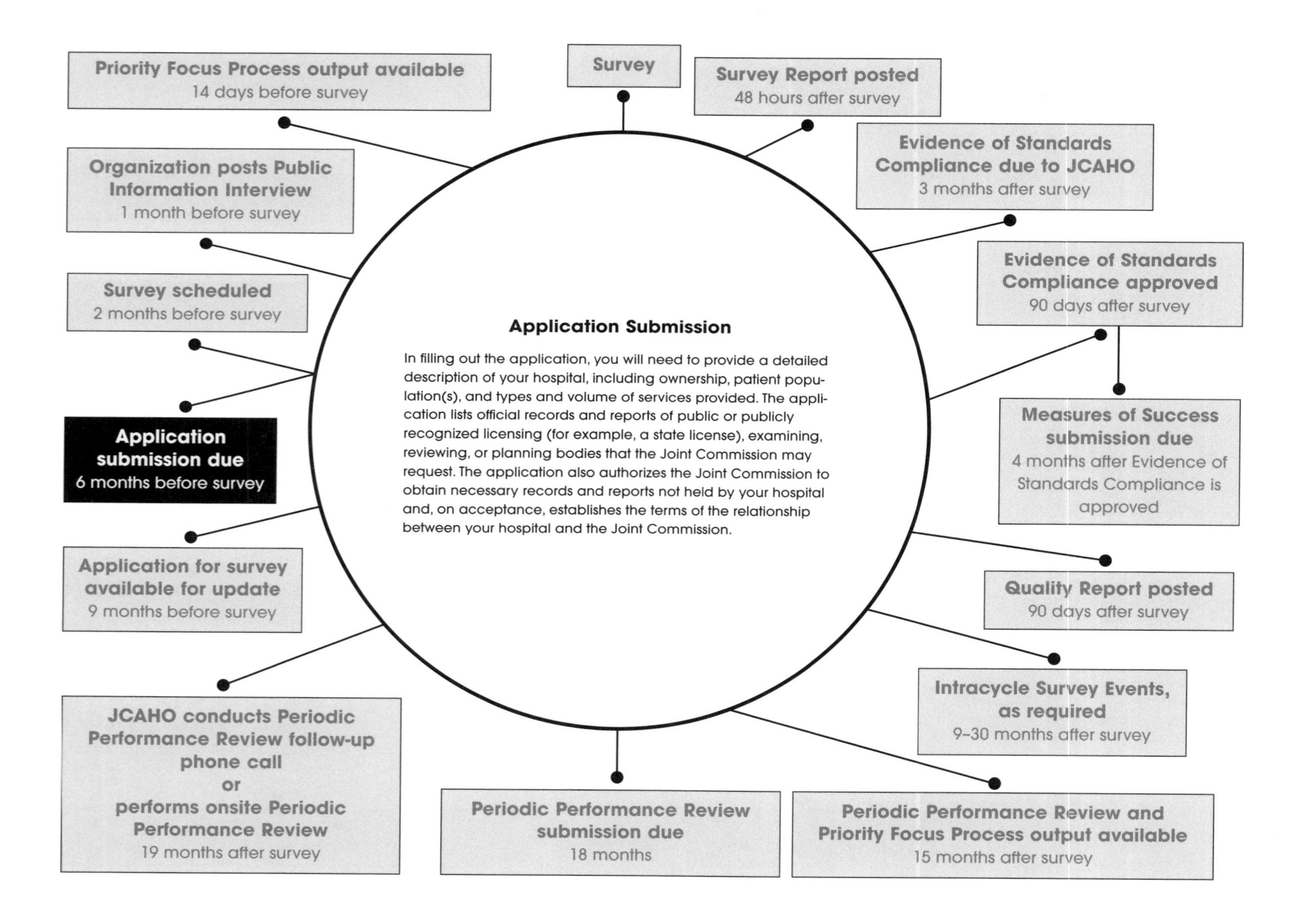
Application for survey available for update
9 months before survey
Application submission due
6 months before survey
Survey scheduled
2 months before survey
Organization posts Public Information Interview
1 month before survey
Priority Focus Process output available
14 days before survey
Survey
Survey Report posted
48 hours after survey
Evidence of Standards Compliance due to JCAHO
3 months after survey
Evidence of Standards Compliance approved
90 days after survey
Measures of Success submission due
4 months after Evidence of Standards Compliance is approved
Quality Report posted
90 days after survey
Intracycle Survey Events, as required
9–30 months after survey
Periodic Performance Review and Priority Focus Process output available
15 months after survey
Periodic Performance Review submission due
18 months
JCAHO conducts Periodic Performance Review follow-up phone call
or
performs onsite Periodic Performance Review
19 months after survey
Application Submission
In filling out the application, you will need to provide a detailed description of your hospital, including ownership, patient population(s), and types and volume of services provided. The application lists official records and reports of public or publicly recognized licensing (for example, a state license), examining, reviewing, or planning bodies that the Joint Commission may request. The application also authorizes the Joint Commission to obtain necessary records and reports not held by your hospital and, on acceptance, establishes the terms of the relationship between your hospital and the Joint Commission.

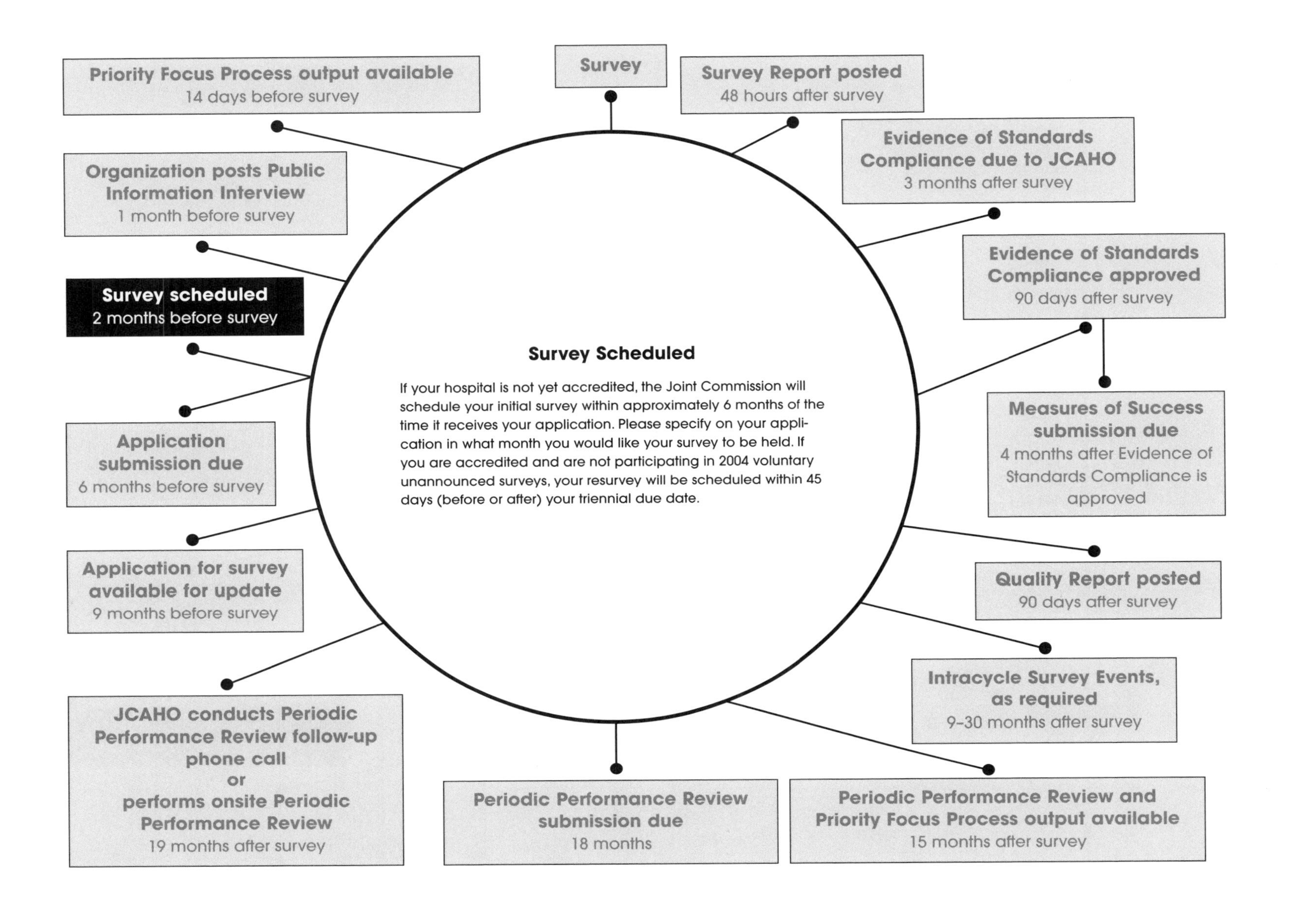
Survey Scheduled
If your hospital is not yet accredited, the Joint Commission will schedule your initial survey within approximately 6 months of the time it receives your application. Please specify on your application in what month you would like your survey to be held. If you are accredited and are not participating in 2004 voluntary unannounced surveys, your resurvey will be scheduled within 45 days (before or after) your triennial due date.
Survey
Survey Report posted
48 hours after survey
Evidence of Standards Compliance due to JCAHO
3 months after survey
Evidence of Standards Compliance approved
90 days after survey
Measures of Success submission due
4 months after Evidence of Standards Compliance is approved
Quality Report posted
90 days after survey
Intracycle Survey Events, as required
9–30 months after survey
Periodic Performance Review and Priority Focus Process output available
15 months after survey
Periodic Performance Review submission due
18 months
JCAHO conducts Periodic Performance Review follow-up phone call
or
performs onsite Periodic Performance Review
19 months after survey
Application for survey available for update
9 months before survey
Application submission due
6 months before survey
Survey scheduled
2 months before survey
Organization posts Public Information Interview
1 month before survey
Priority Focus Process output available
14 days before survey

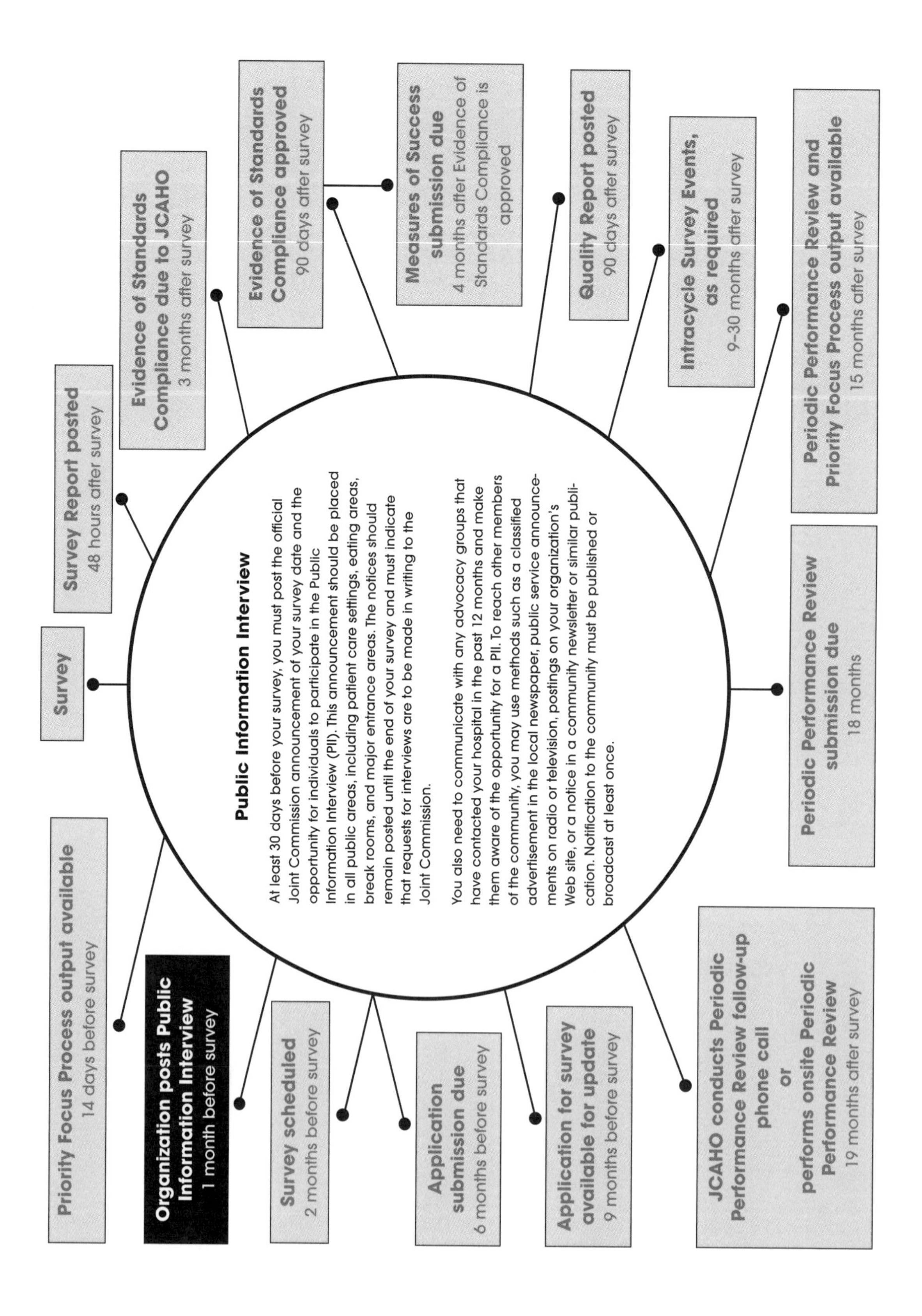
Priority Focus Process output available
14 days before survey
Organization posts Public Information Interview
1 month before survey
Survey scheduled
2 months before survey
Application submission due
6 months before survey
Application for survey available for update
9 months before survey
JCAHO conducts Periodic Performance Review follow-up phone call
or
performs onsite Periodic Performance Review
19 months after survey
Periodic Performance Review submission due
18 months
Periodic Performance Review and Priority Focus Process output available
15 months after survey
Intracycle Survey Events, as required
9–30 months after survey
Quality Report posted
90 days after survey
Measures of Success submission due
4 months after Evidence of Standards Compliance is approved
Evidence of Standards Compliance approved
90 days after survey
Evidence of Standards Compliance due to JCAHO
3 months after survey
Survey Report posted
48 hours after survey
Survey
Public Information Interview
At least 30 days before your survey, you must post the official Joint Commission announcement of your survey date and the opportunity for individuals to participate in the Public Information Interview (PII). This announcement should be placed in all public areas, including patient care settings, eating areas, break rooms, and major entrance areas. The notices should remain posted until the end of your survey and must indicate that requests for interviews are to be made in writing to the Joint Commission.
You also need to communicate with any advocacy groups that have contacted your hospital in the past 12 months and make them aware of the opportunity for a PII. To reach other members of the community, you may use methods such as a classified advertisement in the local newspaper, public service announcements on radio or television, postings on your organization's Web site, or a notice in a community newsletter or similar publication. Notification to the community must be published or broadcast at least once.

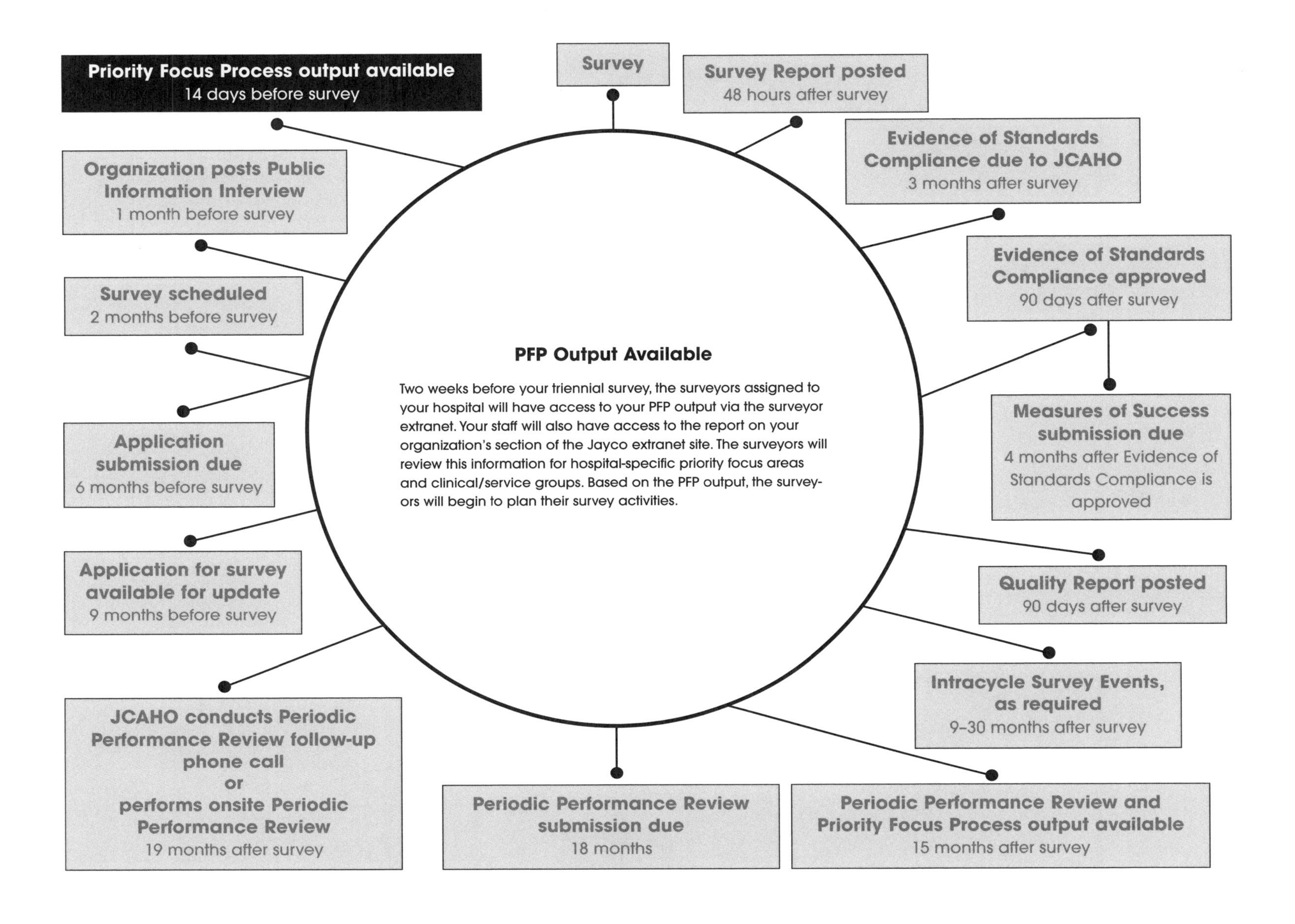
Priority Focus Process output available
14 days before survey
Survey
Survey Report posted
48 hours after survey
Organization posts Public Information Interview
1 month before survey
Evidence of Standards Compliance due to JCAHO
3 months after survey
Survey scheduled
2 months before survey
Evidence of Standards Compliance approved
90 days after survey
PFP Output Available
Two weeks before your triennial survey, the surveyors assigned to your hospital will have access to your PFP output via the surveyor extranet. Your staff will also have access to the report on your organization's section of the Jayco extranet site. The surveyors will review this information for hospital-specific priority focus areas and clinical/service groups. Based on the PFP output, the surveyors will begin to plan their survey activities.
Application submission due
6 months before survey
Measures of Success submission due
4 months after Evidence of Standards Compliance is approved
Application for survey available for update
9 months before survey
Quality Report posted
90 days after survey
Intracycle Survey Events, as required
9–30 months after survey
JCAHO conducts Periodic Performance Review follow-up phone call
or
performs onsite Periodic Performance Review
19 months after survey
Periodic Performance Review submission due
18 months
Periodic Performance Review and Priority Focus Process output available
15 months after survey

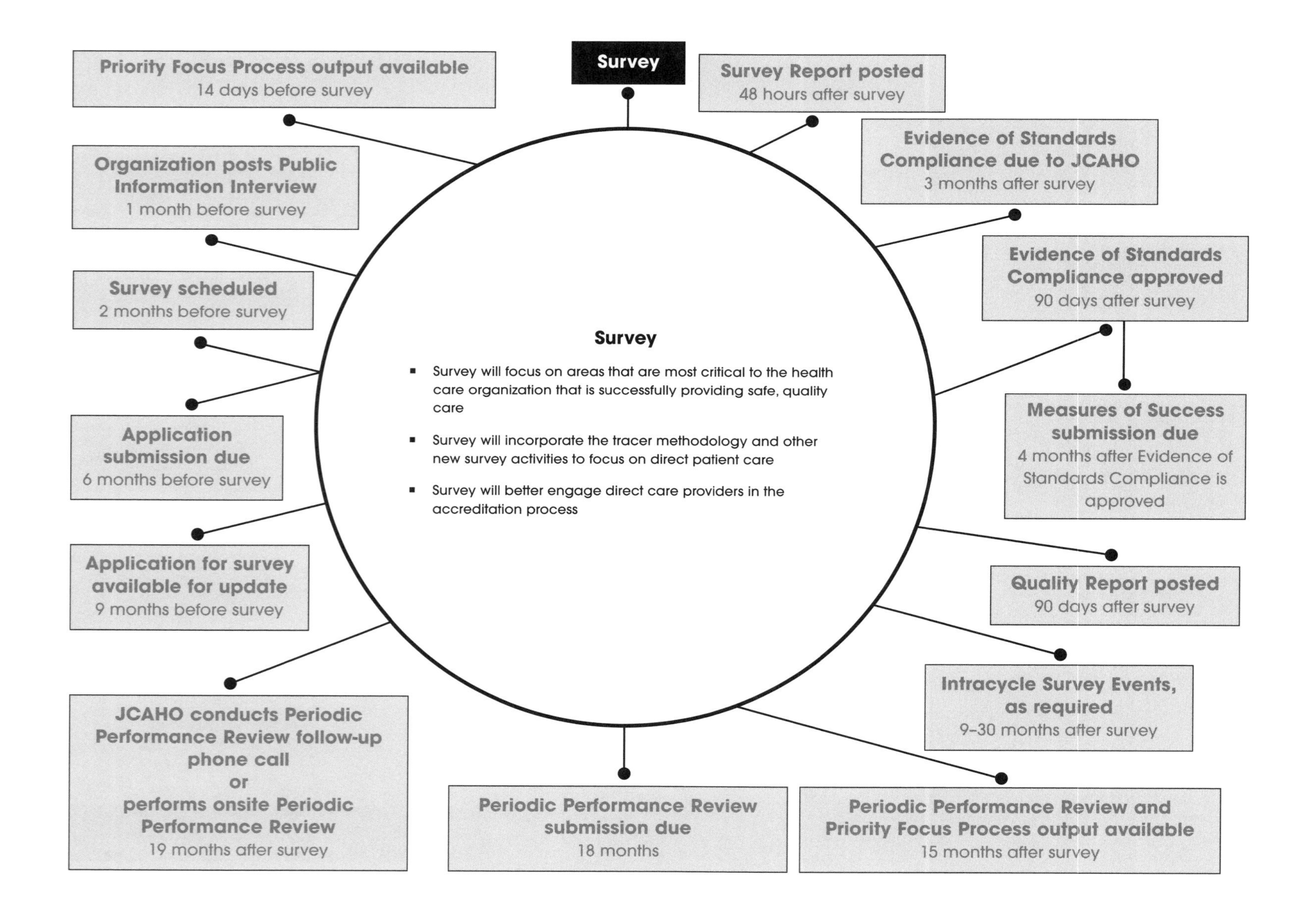

Priority Focus Process output available
14 days before survey
Survey
Survey Report posted
48 hours after survey
Organization posts Public Information Interview
1 month before survey
Evidence of Standards Compliance due to JCAHO
3 months after survey
Survey scheduled
2 months before survey
Evidence of Standards Compliance approved
90 days after survey
Survey
Survey will focus on areas that are most critical to the health care organization that is successfully providing safe, quality care
Survey will incorporate the tracer methodology and other new survey activities to focus on direct patient care
Survey will better engage direct care providers in the accreditation process
Application submission due
6 months before survey
Measures of Success submission due
4 months after Evidence of Standards Compliance is approved
Application for survey available for update
9 months before survey
Quality Report posted
90 days after survey
Intracycle Survey Events, as required
9–30 months after survey
JCAHO conducts Periodic Performance Review follow-up phone call
or
performs onsite Periodic Performance Review
19 months after survey
Periodic Performance Review submission due
18 months
Periodic Performance Review and Priority Focus Process output available
15 months after survey

APPENDIX B

SHARED VISIONS—NEW PATHWAYS FREQUENTLY ASKED QUESTIONS

The Frequently Asked Questions (FAQs) about Shared Visions–New Pathways® included in this appendix are posted to the Joint Commission Web site at http://www.jcaho.org/accredited+organizations/svnp/index.htm. These FAQs are updated frequently by Joint Commission staff and provide a great resource for additional information about the Shared Visions–New Pathways initiative. If your organization has a question about Shared Visions–New Pathways, chances are other organizations have had the same question. So visit the FAQs on the JCAHO Web site whenever you have a question.

If your question is not answered there, you can submit your question to SharedVisions@jcaho.org. Initiative experts will be reviewing these questions and responding accordingly. Your account representative is also a great resource for any information you need as you move through the new accreditation process. As always, standards-specific questions should be directed to the Joint Commission's Standards Interpretation Group at 630/792-5900 or through its online question submission form at http://www.jcaho.org/Onlineform/OnLineForm.asp. Frequently Asked Questions about standards are also included on the Joint Commission Web site.

Overview Questions

When will the new accreditation process be implemented and for which accreditation programs?

The new accreditation process will be implemented beginning in January 2004, with certain components being phased in later for some accreditation programs. Those organizations that will undergo the on-site survey beginning in July 2005 will begin completing the Periodic Performance Review (PPR) in November 2003 (with the exception of the following accreditation programs: assisted living, critical access hospitals, laboratory services, managed behavioral health care, networks, office-based surgery, and preferred provider organizations).

Is the new accreditation process based on new technology?

Yes. JCAHO has developed a secure extranet customer portal, "Jayco"™ Online, to enhance transactions and to process and share information between JCAHO and accredited organizations. One online tool, the e-App, or electronic application for accreditation, was implemented in July 2001, and its ease of use contributes to its growing usage. While the new accreditation process relies heavily on the use of "Jayco"™ Online, paper documents will be accepted.

Will the on-site survey process change?

Yes. The on-site survey will have a tracer methodology, already being introduced in the current survey process, which permits assessment of operational systems and processes in relation to the actual experiences of selected patients who are under the care of the organization. The types of patients selected will be determined by the information provided through the Priority Focus Process (PFP).

Will accreditation decisions remain the same?

No. Beginning in 2004, there will be no scores and accreditation decisions will change. Because of the emphasis on continuous compliance, JCAHO will eliminate the category of Accredited with Requirements for Improvement and will institute new rules for Conditional and Preliminary Denial of Accreditation decisions. As of January 2004, the new accreditation decision categories will be Accredited, Provisional Accreditation, Conditional Accreditation, Preliminary Denial of Accreditation, Denial of Accreditation, and Preliminary Accreditation (under the Early Survey Option).

Will Performance Reports change?

Yes. In July 2004, JCAHO will begin publishing new Quality Reports. The new reports will use symbols—checks, pluses, and minuses—to indicate organization performance and will compare the organization to similar JCAHO–accredited organizations both within the state and nationally. The reports will highlight organization performance related to compliance with JCAHO's National Patient Safety Goals as applicable to the organization, awards and other recognition, and disease-specific care certification among other information. For hospitals, the reports will also show information related to National Quality Goals (ORYX® core measures) and Patient Experience of Care (when this information becomes available). The new Quality Reports will be posted on Quality Check® on JCAHO's Web site.

Complex Organizations

How does the Joint Commission define complex organizations?

A complex organization provides for more than one level and type of health care service, usually in more than one type of setting. Surveying a complex organization involves the use of standards from at least two JCAHO accreditation manuals.

How is JCAHO changing the accreditation process for complex organizations?

JCAHO is making the accreditation process more customized, focused, efficient, and educational for complex organizations. The new survey process will concurrently evaluate all patient/resident/client services throughout the organization in an integrated and seamless manner. Surveyors may survey some standards that apply to multiple programs once across the entire complex organization. For example, one competency assessment process session may involve one surveyor reviewing both home care and hospital human resource files. Surveyors will be assigned, as appropriate, to survey standards applicable only to an individual program.

How does this new pathway compare with the 2003 process for complex organizations?

In previous years for larger complex organizations, surveyors may arrive at an organization at different times to separately survey the services and components of an organization. There's a significant amount of overlap in the standards and survey processes, resulting in some duplication. With the new process, a team of surveyors will survey all of an organization's services and components during a single on-site visit. The focus of the visit will be on how well the organization achieves an integrated approach to patient care.

Why is this a better process for complex organizations?

The new approach will give a truer picture of the flow and integrity of systems throughout the organization's continuum of services. It will allow an organization to see how well linkages are occurring across its services, whether there is a consistent approach to fundamental policies and systems from one component of the organization to another, and how that approach affects patient care.

How does the new approach relate to the tailored survey?

The new approach to surveying larger complex organizations will replace what is now known as the tailored survey, effective January 1, 2004.

How is JCAHO improving the presurvey process for complex organizations?

As part of the new presurvey process, JCAHO will do the following:

- Collect presurvey, detailed information about the organization's specific services and settings from the organization's application for accreditation

- Select a customized set of standards from JCAHO's standards database matched specifically to the organization's characteristics
- Assign credentialed surveyors who have the skills and expertise most appropriate to the organization's characteristics

What kind of accreditation decisions will complex organizations receive?
Complex organizations will continue to receive a comprehensive accreditation decision that reflects the performance of the entire organization. Performance information both at the organization and component levels will continue to be publicly disclosed.

Application for Accreditation

What is the application for accreditation?
The application for accreditation (e-App) gives organizations the option of applying online for accreditation through a secure password protected extranet-site known as "Jayco"™. An accredited organization can access "Jayco"™ six to nine months before its survey due date.

If an organization has never applied for survey before, can it still use the e-App?
Yes. When an organization requests an initial application, it will be sent the User ID and password that will allow data entry in the e-App.

How does an organization use the e-App?
When an organization becomes due for survey, it is provided a password to access the online application on "Jayco"™. The first time an organization logs onto "Jayco"™, it is required to change the password and to submit an e-mail address of the person responsible for access and use of the account.

What is the benefit of using the e-App?
With a paper application, the organization viewed many questions that were not pertinent to its setting. The e-App contains screening questions that help focus and reduce the total amount of questions that must be asked. In addition, the data will be stored for the user so once the e-App has been filled out, much of the information from the previous application can simply be reviewed and updated. Using the e-App results in more accurate application information and fewer phone calls between the organization and JCAHO—a big time saver. Multiple users can work on an organization's e-App simultaneously.

Will my organization have to spend a lot of time searching for information specific to my organization?
No, you will only see the screens that you need for the services your organization provides.

What are the technical requirements for using the e-App?
The 2003 (e-App) requires using Microsoft Internet Explorer browser release 5.0 or higher.

How secure is the "Jayco"™ section of the Web site?
JCAHO understands that security is important and we have taken steps to ensure that your organization's information is protected. First, access is restricted to accredited organizations or to those organizations seeking accreditation for the first time. We require all users to have a valid login ID and password to gain access to "Jayco"™. Once an organization's information is received, it is stored behind a firewall—a security system that prevents unauthorized access to or from a private network. Only users to whom the organization has assigned a login ID and password will have access to its information.

Whom do I call if I have questions about the e-App?
Individual health care organizations should call their account representative at 630/792-3007. Corporate organizations participating in our multistate programs can contact their account representative at his or her direct extension. Account representatives are trained to walk you through the process. Or send an e-mail to jaycofeedback@jcaho.org.

On-Site Survey Process

Why is the survey process changing?
The survey process is being substantially modified to enhance its value, relevance, and credibility. The process will be data-driven and patient-centered and will have a greater focus on evaluating the organization's processes of care.

What are the benefits of the new survey agenda?

- More time for the surveyors to concentrate on the issues most important to each organization surveyed
- A survey process customized to the organization's settings, services, patient population, and demographics
- More focus given to the delivery of care (guided by the Priority Focus Process [PFP] and tracer methodology)
- Fewer formal interviews
- Reduced paperwork and burden of preparing documentation for survey

How will surveyors be retrained to effectively perform Shared Visions–New Pathways surveys?
Beginning at the January 2003 Annual Surveyor Conference and continuing throughout 2003 via distance learning, surveyors are receiving education and testing in systems theory, organization behavior, and evaluation techniques under a program administered by the Kellogg School of Management at Northwestern

University. In addition, surveyors and their supervisors started receiving aggregated performance data in 2003. These internal management reports allow supervisors to track data by surveyor and in the aggregate. This reporting creates another quality control mechanism, and it also helps to identify areas for future surveyor development.

How will the new survey process be more consistently applied and be more organization-specific?

The PFP lends consistency to the surveyor's on-site sampling process by helping surveyors evaluate presurvey data consistently for all health care organizations. By using the PFP, the survey process also becomes more customized to the specific characteristics of the organization being accredited. In addition, by using the tracer methodology, surveyors will evaluate the services that a specific organization provides, as well as the interaction of departments and functions throughout the organization.

Performance Measurement

How will performance measurement data, such as ORYX® and core measures, fit into Shared Visions–New Pathways?

Performance measurement data are an integral part of Shared Visions–New Pathways. JCAHO will be using data as a mechanism to help steer surveyors toward areas within an organization that the data suggest might represent important performance improvement opportunities. Similarly, surveyors may also use these data to identify areas where organization performance is above average, indicating that organizations may be candidates for JCAHO's good practices database. Data will also form the focus of discussion between the surveyor and the organization with respect to performance improvement and how the organization is using data to continuously improve its processes of care.

Will ORYX® and core measure requirements for hospitals change as a result of Shared Visions–New Pathways?

Changes in the core measure requirements for hospitals coincide with the implementation of Shared Visions–New Pathways on January 1, 2004, but are not a direct result of the new accreditation process. JCAHO's Board of Commissioners approved the implementation of requirements for a third core measure set for the hospital program. So, hospitals with appropriate services currently collecting two of four measure sets—for example, acute myocardial infarction, heart failure, community-acquired pneumonia—and pregnancy and related conditions will be required to collect three of four measure sets.

Will performance measurement requirements change for ambulatory care, behavioral health care, home care, or long term care organizations?

With respect to these accreditation programs, nothing will change relative to performance measurement requirements with the implementation of Shared

Visions–New Pathways, whether the organization is collecting core measures or noncore measures. Over time, as JCAHO develops additional core measures, it is likely that requirements may be added; however, in the initial phases of the new accreditation process, there will be no changes for these accreditation programs.

How will the new accreditation process be more data driven?
Through the PFP, a variety of data inputs will be used to help guide the on-site survey process. MedPAR data (collected by the Centers for Medicare & Medicaid Services), sentinel event data, ORYX® core measure data, complaint data, and pertinent demographic data from the organization will be factored into a rules-driven process to identify areas for focus during the on-site survey.

How will surveyors use ORYX® and core measure data in the new accreditation process?
Both now and in the future, surveyors have access to ORYX® data. Surveyors receive a presurvey report that summarizes information on the measures the organization is using. For accreditation programs without core measures, surveyors receive reports on the noncore measure data and the actual performance results. Surveyors converse with organization staff to find out how they are using data in their performance improvement activities.

How will performance measurement data be reflected in JCAHO's Quality Reports?
ORYX® and core measure data will be a significant component of JCAHO's Quality Reports. JCAHO is currently working on a format for these reports that will translate the data into information that is understandable and meaningful to the various stakeholders and individuals who will rely on it.

Periodic Performance Review

What is the Periodic Performance Review?
The Periodic Performance Review (PPR) is a new form of evaluation that is conducted at the midpoint of the accreditation cycle and focuses on patient safety and quality-of-care issues. Under the full PPR, the organization self-evaluates its compliance with all standards and elements of performance (EPs) (scoreable requirements) that are applicable to the services that the organization provides and develops a plan of action for all areas of performance identified as needing improvement. JCAHO will work with the organization to refine its plan(s) of action to assure that the organization's improvement efforts are on target. The organization will also identify measures of success (MOS) for validating resolution of the identified problem areas when the organization undergoes its complete on-site survey 18 months later.

Is there an option to conducting the PPR?
Yes. In response to concerns about legal disclosure of PPR information shared with JCAHO, three options to the full PPR are available to organizations. The options and their requirements are as follows:

Option 1

- The organization performs the midcycle self-assessment and develops the plan(s) of action and MOS but does not submit PPR data to JCAHO
- The organization affirms that it has completed the foregoing activities but has, for substantive reasons, been advised not to submit its self-assessment or plan(s) of action to JCAHO
- The organization may discuss standards-related issues with JCAHO staff without identifying its specific levels of standards compliance
- At the time of the complete on-site survey, the organization provides its MOS to JCAHO for assessment

Option 2

- The organization does not conduct a midcycle self-assessment
- The organization undergoes an on-site survey at the midpoint of its accreditation cycle. The survey will be approximately one-third the length of a typical full on-site survey, and the organization will be charged a fee to cover survey costs.
- The organization develops and submits to JCAHO a plan of action to address any areas of noncompliance found during the on-site survey. JCAHO will work with the organization to refine its plan of action.
- At the time of the complete on-site survey, the organization provides its MOS to JCAHO for assessment

Option 3

- The organization does not conduct a midcycle self-assessment
- The organization undergoes an on-site survey at the midpoint of its accreditation cycle. The survey will be approximately one-third the length of a typical full on-site survey, and the organization will be charged a fee to cover survey costs.
- At the time of the complete on-site survey, the surveyors will receive no information relating to the organization's option 3 survey findings

What are the benefits of conducting a full PPR versus one of the options?
Both the full PPR and the options facilitate a more continuous accreditation process by incorporating an additional form of evaluation. The full PPR has the additional benefit of helping to ensure consistency in accreditation because the scoring methodology for the PPR is the same as that used by surveyors during the on-site survey.

How does the plan of action affect my organization's accreditation decision?
If the plan of action is approved, the organization's accreditation decision will remain the same. However, if the plan of action is not approved, the organization's accreditation decision will be changed to reflect the appropriate status. At the triennial on-site survey, implementation of the plan of action will be validated.

How do I complete my organization's PPR or indicate that I have selected an option?
The full PPR, or the selection of an option to the full PPR, is completed and submitted to JCAHO electronically, using JCAHO's secure extranet customer portal called "Jayco"™. If you select an option, the electronic tool automatically provides a screen with the attestation and instructions on how to complete it. Each accredited organization receives a password and user ID that allows them secure access to "Jayco"™. "Jayco"™ is protected by "firewalls" that block access to users who do not have correct passwords and/or user IDs. "Jayco"™ enhances transactions as well as the processing and sharing of information between JCAHO and accredited organizations in a secure environment.

When do we need to conduct the PPR or select an option?
Either the full PPR or the selection of option 1 or option 2 needs to be completed and submitted 18 months after the last survey.

How does the full PPR and options fit into the new accreditation process?
JCAHO's new accreditation process, Shared Visions–New Pathways, is designed to help organizations maintain continuous compliance with the standards, and use them as a management tool for doing business and improving patient care and safety. The PPR and the options provide the framework for continuous standards compliance and focus on the critical systems and process that affect patient care and safety.

Priority Focus Process

What is the Priority Focus Process?
The Priority Focus Process (PFP) is a data-driven tool that helps focus survey activity on issues most relevant to patient safety and quality of care at the specific health care organization being surveyed.

How does the PFP fit into the new accreditation process?

The PFP uses automation to gather presurvey data from multiple sources including the Joint Commission, the health care organization, and other public sources. The PFP then applies rules to 1) identify relevant standards and appropriate survey activities and 2) guide the selection of patient tracers. (As part of the PFP, surveyors will track patients, residents, or clients through their experience of care within an organization, assessing the quality and safety of care provided.) The PFP does not imply that priority areas are out of compliance or deficient in any way; rather, it lends consistency to the surveyor's on-site sampling process.

Why will the PFP improve the accreditation process?

By providing presurvey information to surveys which has been developed using a standardized methodology, the PFP will help surveyors evaluate health care organizations' performance more consistently. The PFP also helps to focus the surveyors' assessment on quality and safety issues specific to an individual health care organization.

What kind of organization-specific information will the PFP identify?

The output of the PFP process will include the following:

- The top four to five priority focus areas (PFAs)—the processes, systems, or structures within a health care organization known to significantly impact the safety and quality of care specific to the health care organization being surveyed
- The clinical/service groups—groups of patients, residents, or clients in distinct clinical populations for which data are collected. For example, in a hospital setting, clinical/service groups might include cardiology, general surgery, or orthopedic and rehabilitation. In an ambulatory setting, clinical/service groups could include gastroenterology, obstetrics, and pediatrics.

Information from the priority focus areas and clinical/service groups will then be used to help guide the focus of the on-site survey activities.

When will an organization have access to its priority focus information?

The information will be sent to health care organizations along with its access to the extranet-based PPR approximately 15 months after their last triennial survey and then again 1 to 2 weeks prior to their on-site survey, when the information is also shared with surveyors.

Quality Report

What are Quality Reports?

The Joint Commission has had a longstanding commitment to providing meaningful information about the comparative performance of accredited organizations to the public. JCAHO began publishing organization–specific Performance Reports in 1994. As part of the Joint Commission's Shared Visions–New Pathways initiative, JCAHO will publish an enhanced version of Performance Reports called Quality Reports beginning in the third quarter of 2004. The new Quality Reports will provide consumers with relevant and useful information about the quality and safety of JCAHO–accredited organizations.

What will the new Quality Reports look like?

The new reports will feature a user-friendly format with checks, pluses, and minuses to help consumers compare health care organization performance in a number of key areas. The performance of organizations accredited after January 1, 2004, will be reported under the new Quality Report format.

What will happen to Performance Reports?

Historical Performance Reports will continue to be available after the implementation of Quality Reports. Performance Reports will be generated for all 2003 surveys. Performance Reports are available in Quality Check® at http://www.jcaho.org.

What information will be available in the Quality Reports?

The improved reports will provide the following information about a health care organization:

- JCAHO accreditation status and the effective dates of the accreditation award. If an organization has Provisional Accreditation status, the standards in which the organization is lacking compliance will be listed. This information is not immediately available; the organization has 90 days (45 days beginning July 1, 2005) following the survey to submit Evidence of Standards Compliance (ESC).
- Compliance with JCAHO's National Patient Safety Goals, as applicable to the organization. JCAHO established goals to help accredited organizations address specific areas of concern in regards to patient safety. The Quality Report contains the goals in effect at the time of an organization's survey and reports if an organization has successfully implemented the goals or an acceptable alternative. The goals are listed with an explanation of the method to achieve the goal. For example, goal #1 "Improve the accuracy of patient identification" is listed with the requirement to "Use at least two patient identifiers when taking blood or administering medication." Implementation of the goals and the associated recommendation is denoted by a checkmark. If the goal or requirement is not applicable to the organization, the report will show an NA for "Not Applicable." Goals

that have not been implemented and have resulted in an open Requirement for Improvement will not have a checkmark.

- Performance on National Quality Improvement Goals (ORYX® core measures, for hospitals only). National Quality Improvement Goals allow hospitals to report on the key indicators of quality of care in three of four treatment areas: heart attack, heart failure, community acquired pneumonia, and pregnancy and related conditions. Algorithms are used to determine if an organization's performance is above, similar to, or below the performance of other JCAHO–accredited organizations. Comparative analysis is done at a state level and nationwide. In addition to reporting results at a measurement level (for example, "aspirin at arrival"), comparative results are calculated at a measurement set level (for example, heart attack). This information is converted to an easy-to-understand "at-a-glance" representation of performance along with supporting detailed results and numerical ranges. The comparative results are recalculated on an ongoing basis using the most recent four quarters of measurement results.
- Patient experience of care information (for hospitals only). This information is derived from a voluntary reporting initiative developed by the Centers for Medicare & Medicaid Services (CMS). It covers key patient care issues. As this information is made available, it will be included in the Quality Reports.
- Quality distinctions, including recognition such as Disease-Specific Care Certification, Ernest A. Codman Award, and Magnet status (awarded by the American Nurses Credentialing Center), among others

Who provided input on the new Quality Reports?

JCAHO proactively sought input from consumers regarding the form and content of accreditation information that would be useful to them. A series of feedback sessions was held across the country involving a variety of socio-economic groups to ensure that the new Quality Reports meet public expectations. In addition, JCAHO sought advice from its program–specific advisory groups, business leaders, health care experts, and consumer advocates.

When will Quality Reports become available to the public?

The performance of health care organizations receiving an award of accreditation during 2004 will be reported in the new Quality Report format. The revised reports are expected to be available on the JCAHO Web site at Quality Check® beginning in the third quarter of 2004. Certain components of the reports will be provided as information becomes available. In 2004, the National Patient Safety Goal results for hospitals that are surveyed in 2003 and 2004 and the Quality Improvement Goal results for all hospitals will be available. The performance of accredited organizations will continue to be reported in the Performance Report format until the organization becomes reaccredited, at which time its performance will be reflected on the new Quality Reports.

Scoring and Accreditation Decisions

Why is the Joint Commission changing its accreditation decision process?

JCAHO's previous accreditation decision process was a multilayered, score-based system. The new accreditation decision process does the following:

- Reflects Shared Visions–New Pathways' focus on ongoing standards compliance
- Is more credible, assuring the public that accredited organizations have demonstrated full compliance with the standards
- Is based primarily on the number of standards that are scored not compliant
- Simplifies the compliance screening process in determining an accreditation decision. The "grid" score is eliminated, and standards are scored on a three-point scale instead of a five-point scale.
- Focuses less on "scores" and more on using the standards to achieve and maintain excellent operational systems

Do certain elements of performance have more weight in the new process?

No. However, it is important to note that standards are scored based on a percentage of their elements of performance (EP) that are scored insufficient compliance or partial compliance. Some standards may have only one EP, while other standards have more.

Does a single EP scored 0 (insufficient compliance) or 1 (partial compliance) automatically trigger a not compliant standard?

Not necessarily. If a single EP under a given standard is scored 0 (insufficient compliance), then that standard would be scored 0 (not compliant). However, 35% or more of the EPs under a specific standard would have to be scored 1 (partially compliant) for that standard to be considered not compliant.

What happens if standards are scored not compliant?

If standards are scored not compliant at the time of the on-site survey, an organization must demonstrate that it has corrected systems and processes to be in compliance with those standards by submitting Evidence of Standards Compliance (ESC). From January 2004 through June 2005, organizations will have 90 days to submit an ESC to JCAHO because they will not have the benefit of completing a PPR and identifying standards that are not compliant prior to the on-site survey. After June 2005, organizations will have 45 days to submit an ESC to JCAHO because the PPR will be available to them. In addition to the ESC, the organization will also submit an indicator or MOS that it will use to assess sustained compliance over time. Four months after approval of the ESC, the organization will submit data on its MOS to demonstrate sustained compliance over time.

Will health care organizations receive an overall score?

There will be no overall score or grid element score with the new accreditation decision process, and no scores will be shared with the health care organization. However, the Accreditation Report will list requirements for improvement by priority focus area. The Accreditation Report will include the standard number, the text of the standard, the specific findings of the survey team, and the EPs that are partially compliant or insufficiently compliant. The organization must address all requirements for improvement, in the form of ESC, to be accredited. The Accreditation Report will also include supplemental findings, which are situations where EPs were scored partially compliant but did not cause the standard to be scored not compliant. Supplemental findings do not require an ESC to be submitted.

How are the accreditation decision categories changing?

If an organization demonstrates compliance with all of the standards at the time of the on-site survey, or resolves requirements for improvement via an acceptable ESC submission, it will receive a decision of ***Accredited.*** Because of the emphasis on continuous compliance, JCAHO eliminated the category of Accredited with Requirements for Improvement and has instituted new rules for Conditional and Preliminary Denial of Accreditation decisions. If an organization is not in compliance, it will receive one of the following accreditation decisions (the following are not official definitions, but explanations):

- ***Provisional Accreditation*** - All requirements for improvement have not been addressed in the ESC submission, or the organization has failed to achieve an appropriate level of sustained compliance as determined by an MOS result
- ***Conditional Accreditation*** - Number of standards scored not compliant is between two and three standard deviations above the mean number of not compliant standards for organizations in that accreditation program. The organization must undergo an on-site follow-up survey.
- ***Preliminary Denial of Accreditation*** - Number of standards scored not compliant is three or more standard deviations above the mean number of not compliant standards for organizations in that accreditation program. There is justification to deny accreditation, but the decision is subject to appeal.
- ***Denial of Accreditation*** - The organization has been denied accreditation, and all review and appeal opportunities have been exhausted
- ***Preliminary Accreditation*** - The organization demonstrates compliance with selected standards in the first of two surveys conducted under the Early Survey Policy Option 1. This decision remains in effect until one of the other official accreditation decision categories is assigned, based on a complete survey against all applicable standards approximately six months later.

When will organizations receive their final accreditation decisions?
Following the survey, surveyors will leave an Accreditation Report on-site. However, the final accreditation decision will be made after JCAHO receives and approves an organization's ESC submission and its MOS. If an acceptable ESC is received, then the organization will receive a decision of Accredited.

Standards Review Project

What is the Standards Review Project?
Launched in 2000 by the Joint Commission, the Standards Review Project involved a sweeping review of all of the standards for all of JCAHO's accreditation programs (excluding assisted living, critical access hospitals, networks, and office-based surgery), and of the requirements for demonstrating compliance with the standards.

Why did JCAHO conduct a comprehensive standards review?
JCAHO has added standards over the years to address emerging quality and safety challenges and to maintain a set of state-of-the-art standards. However, JCAHO had not completed a comprehensive review of the relevance of all standards since the Agenda for Change in the early 1990s. The objectives of the Standards Review Project are to do the following:

- Reduce the number of standards by eliminating standards that are no longer relevant to safe, high quality care
- Improve the clarity and relevance of the remaining standards. As appropriate, the standards have a rationale that describes the standard's purpose and background.
- Reduce the paperwork and documentation burden associated with demonstrating compliance with standards
- Align the standards requirements—now known as Elements of Performance (EPs)—with surveyor assessment and scoring protocols. This alignment ensures that the same expectations used by the surveyors are available to organizations.
- Ensure consistency between accreditation programs. This consistency eases compliance requirements for complex organizations—those accredited under more than one program.

Are the 2004 standards new?
No. The resulting standards are not new; the modifications represent deletions, consolidations, or clarifications of existing standards. However, in parallel projects—for example, Medication Management—new requirements have been added. In addition, some EPs that existed in one manual may now be applicable across all manuals, so there may be new expectations in some manuals.

When will the standards become effective and for what programs do they apply?

The revised standards become effective on January 1, 2004. The standards apply to the ambulatory, behavioral health care, home care, hospital, laboratory, and long term care programs.

Who reviewed the standards?

A special Standards Review Task Force, a Medical Staff Chapter Task Force, and an Information Management Task Force were formed to conduct a thorough review of the standards. In the spring of 2002, the external review process for the proposed revised standards for the various accreditation programs began. The proposed standards were distributed in a field engagement to selected JCAHO accredited organizations and were submitted for review and comment to JCAHO advisory groups, including each accreditation program's Professional and Technical Advisory Committee. The proposed revised standards have been reviewed and approved by JCAHO's Standards and Survey Procedures Committee and JCAHO's Board of Commissioners.

What are the benefits of the Standards Review Project?

The revised standards are the foundation of JCAHO's new accreditation process, Shared Visions–New Pathways. This new process is designed to help organizations maintain continuous compliance with the standards and use them as a management tool for doing business and improving patient care and safety. The Standards Review Project resulted in improved relevance and clarity of the standards and the associated EPs. The number of standards was reduced significantly—for example, by 56% in the hospital program.

Surveyor Development

What is JCAHO doing to improve surveyor skills?

A large component of the new survey process focuses on systems analysis, which depends on a thorough and credible evaluation. Therefore, it is critical that surveyors provide flexible, yet consistent and accurate standards compliance interpretation. To encourage this, JCAHO is certifying surveyors, a process that includes implementing formal, systems analysis training; observing surveyors during actual surveys on an announced and unannounced basis; and measuring and tracking surveyor performance.

Why is surveyor certification important?

Because of the importance of surveyors in directly interacting with health care organizations, JCAHO places the utmost importance on continuously developing its surveyor cadre and monitoring the competence of its surveyors in the field. The introduction of the Surveyor Certification Examination in January 2002 was an important example of this commitment. JCAHO is the first—and only—accrediting body to certify its surveyors this way.

What type of training are surveyors receiving?

Beginning at the January 2003 Annual Surveyor Conference and continuing throughout 2003 via distance learning, surveyors received education and testing in systems theory, organization behavior, and evaluation techniques under a program administered by the Kellogg School of Management at Northwestern University.

Are surveyors being monitored and observed?

Yes. Starting in January 2002, surveyor supervisors and mentors began observing surveyors in the field on both an announced and unannounced basis to further support surveyor skill development. JCAHO managers observe surveyors during actual surveys. In addition, surveyors-in-training must observe certified surveyors conducting on-site evaluations.

How is surveyor performance being measured and tracked?

Surveyors and their supervisors started receiving aggregated performance data in 2003. These internal management reports allow supervisors to track data by surveyor and in the aggregate. This report creates another quality control mechanism, and it also serves to identify areas for future surveyor development.

Tracer Methodology

What is the tracer methodology?

Tracer methodology is an evaluation method that uses a medical/clinical record as a way to evaluate an organization's performance of care and services provided as viewed and experienced by the patient, resident, and client and as provided and coordinated by your organization.

How will surveyors use tracers to assess care and safety?

Using tracers, JCAHO surveyors will look at the care provided by each department within an organization and how departments work together. Surveyors retrace the specific care processes that the individual experienced by observing and talking to staff in areas that the individual received care.

What will surveyors be looking for?

As the individual's case is examined, the surveyor may identify performance issues in one or more steps of the process—or the interfaces between steps—that affect the care of the patient, resident, or client. Surveyors will look for commonalities that might point to potential system-level issues in the organization. The tracer activity also provides several opportunities for surveyors to provide education to organization staff and leaders, as well as to share best practices from other similar health care organizations.

How will individuals be selected as tracers?

Tracer patients, residents, or clients will be selected primarily from an active patient list. Typically, individuals selected for the tracer activity are those who have received multiple or complex services.

How many tracers will be completed at each organization?
The number of tracers completed depends on the length of the survey; however, the average three-day hospital survey with a team of three surveyors typically allows for completion of approximately 11 tracers.

Will surveyors speak to tracer patients?
As in the current survey process, the surveyor may speak to the patient, resident, or client during the tracer activity, if it is appropriate. As always, the surveyor asks for patient permission before speaking to him or her.

What happens if surveyors identify a problem trend at an organization?
If problem trends are identified, surveyors will issue the organization a requirement for improvement. From January 1, 2004, to July 1, 2005, the organization has 90 days from the end of the survey to submit ESC and identify MOS that it will use to assess sustained compliance over time. After July 1, 2005, the organization will have 45 days from the end of the survey to submit ESC and identify MOS. Four months after approval of the ESC, the organization will submit data on its MOS to demonstrate a track record. Any exchange of information between the health care organization and the Joint Commission will meet HIPAA requirements.

Unannounced Survey Process

Why is the Joint Commission shifting from announced surveys to unannounced surveys?
The Joint Commission will be implementing unannounced surveys to accomplish the following:

- Enhance the credibility of the accreditation process by ensuring that surveyors observe the performance of an organization under normal circumstances
- Reduce the unnecessary costs that health care organizations may incur to prepare for survey
- Address public concerns that the Joint Commission receive an accurate reflection of the quality and safety of care
- Help health care organizations focus on providing safe, high quality care at all times, not just when preparing for survey

When will unannounced surveys take effect?
The Joint Commission's Board of Commissioner's approved a proposal to conduct all regular accreditation surveys on an unannounced basis beginning in January 2006.

How do unannounced surveys fit into the new accreditation process?
JCAHO's new accreditation process, Shared Visions–New Pathways, is designed to help organizations maintain continuous compliance with the standards and use them as a management tool for doing business and improving patient care and safety. Shared Visions–New Pathways sets the stage for unannounced surveys that will ensure that the observation and assessment of the organization's patient care processes are performed without any special preparation for the on-site survey.

What kind of field input is JCAHO seeking on unannounced surveys?
JCAHO will work closely with its various advisory groups, accredited organizations, and other stakeholder groups to gain their input and smooth the transition to unannounced surveys.

How will JCAHO test the unannounced survey model?
The transition to unannounced surveys will begin with pilot tests conducted in volunteer organizations during 2004 and 2005. Beginning in 2004, JCAHO will pilot test the unannounced survey process in all types of accredited organizations. During that time, small but important modifications to the on-site survey process will be tested to accommodate organization staff who may be absent or unavailable when surveyors arrive for an unannounced survey. These modifications will prevent such an occurrence from causing any disadvantage to the organization or to the surveyor. In addition, feedback from the pilot tests may also result in other changes to the current unannounced survey process model.

Will JCAHO continue to conduct random unannounced surveys?
Through the end of 2006, JCAHO plans to continue to conduct one-day random, unannounced surveys in an annual 5% sample of the health care organizations it accredits.

How will JCAHO survey organizations seeking accreditation for the first time?
Initial surveys for organizations seeking accreditation for the first time will continue to be conducted on an announced basis.

APPENDIX C

TALKING POINTS FOR THE NEW ACCREDITATION PROCESS

In this appendix you will find information you can share with your governing body, medical staff, employees, and other key audiences about your survey.

Remind your audiences of the following:

- Shared Visions–New Pathways® is an entirely new approach to evaluating quality and safety in your organization
- Shared Visions–New Pathways shifts the view of accreditation—it is no longer a snapshot. It is a feature-length film, providing panoramic insight into your organization's daily operations and systems.
- The new accreditation process makes the process you have just undergone a true validation of the organization's continuous improvement efforts
- The emphasis on continuous improvement efforts carries over into sharing information about the results of the on-site survey
- A final accreditation decision will be made after Joint Commission staff review and approve the health care organization's ESC (Evidence of Standards Compliance) and any identified MOS (measure of success). The Central Office review is completed within 30 days of receiving the ESC. If the health care organization successfully addresses all of its improvement requirements, the organization will be Accredited. This final decision will be posted on the Joint Commission's Web site, http://www.jcaho.org, beginning in the third quarter of 2004. If some of the improvement requirements are not resolved, your organization will be Provisionally Accredited.
- Upon receipt of its accreditation award, the health care organization may publicly disclose the survey decision and any findings

With this process come the following new measures of success:

- Focus on successfully achieving accreditation, which is recognized nationally as the Gold Seal of Approval™ in health care
- Focus on the fact that you have undergone a thorough on-site review and are committed to meeting rigorous national standards—continuously. The conclusion of the new accreditation process is a validation of the work to continuously comply with standards in the weeks and months ahead.
- Emphasize your public commitment to continuous improvement and delivering safe, high-quality care
- Stress how ongoing compliance with Joint Commission standards results in sound management practices in the daily delivery of high-quality and safe care. The Joint Commission survey serves as an independent audit of your organization's commitment to continuous quality improvement.
- Share information specific to your organization about what accreditation means by, for example, detailing your full compliance with particular areas of the accreditation process, such as challenging standards, or your level of compliance with 250 standards (for hospitals)
- Emphasize your compliance with National Patient Safety Goals
- Demonstrate your successful performance by sharing your ORYX® data or national improvement goals (for hospitals), or OASIS data (for home care organizations) or MDS data (for long term care organizations)
- Stress your focus on continuous standards compliance over the course of the three-year accreditation cycle (rather than once every three years) and point out the fact that efforts to maintain a constant state of survey readiness improve the safety and care of patients, residents, and clients—the ultimate aim of accreditation
- Compare systems issues they identified during the Periodic Performance Review (PPR) process with the on-site survey findings and emphasize the improvements made as a result of this ongoing work
- If organizations have ESC and MOS requirements, you may want to share information about these improvement efforts. Leadership might, for example, compare this process to a financial audit by an accounting firm in which organizations have an opportunity either to present evidence contrary to the auditors' findings or to accept the report and implement improvement strategies.
- Use specific examples of staff and physician involvement in the accreditation process and satisfaction with that involvement to demonstrate a measure of success
- Discuss how staff involvement was vital to the on-site survey because of the focus on patient care through the tracer methodology and observation of care
- Emphasize how the accreditation survey is now tailored to each organization's unique characteristics and services

GLOSSARY

Accreditation Report
A report of an organization's survey findings; the report includes requirements for improvement and supplemental findings, as appropriate.

Application for accreditation (e-App)
Form used for collecting information pertaining to the requestor organization. Information collected on this form will be used to determine the accreditation standards applicable to the organization, the types of surveyors needed, the length of the survey, and the survey fee. Information concerning all applicable accreditation programs, with the exception of laboratory services, is to be included in a single Application for Survey form for each organization. To obtain JCAHO accreditation for laboratory services, a separate Application for Accreditation for laboratory accreditation is required.

Clinical/service groups (CSGs)
Groups of clients, residents, or patients in distinct clinical populations for which data are collected. Tracer subjects are selected according to CSGs.

Element(s) of Performance (EP or EPs)
A specific performance expectation with reference to a standard which details the specific structures, processes, or systems that must be in place for an organization to provide quality care, treatment, and services. Compliance with a single EP, or more typically multiple EPs, will determine compliance with the intent of a standard. EPs are scored on a three-point scale: 0 = Unsatisfactory Compliance, 1 = Partial Compliance, and 2 = Satisfactory Compliance.

Evidence of Standards Compliance (ESC)
A report submitted by a surveyed organization within 45 days* of its survey,

which details the action(s) that it took to bring itself into compliance with a standard or clarifies why the organization says that it was in compliance with the standard for which it received a recommendation. An ESC must address compliance at the element of performance (EP) level and include a measure of success for all appropriate EP corrections.
* From January 1, 2004, through July 1, 2005, this time frame for submission of the ESC will be extended to 90 days.

Full Periodic Performance Review (PPR)
An additional requirement of the accreditation process whereby an organization reviews its compliance with all applicable JCAHO standards; completes and submits to JCAHO a plan of action for any standard not in full compliance, including the identification of a measure of success (MOS); and engages in a telephone discussion with a member of the Standards Interpretation Group staff to determine the acceptability of the plan of action. The PPR will encourage organizations to be in continuous compliance with JCAHO standards. Surveyors will see an organization's plan of action to validate that the MOS were effective.

"Jayco"™
"Jayco"™ is a secure, password-protected Web site for information from and communication with JCAHO for accredited organizations and key stakeholders.

Measure(s) of success (MOS)
A numerical or quantifiable measure usually related to an audit that determines if an action was effective and sustained. An MOS report is due four months after the Evidence of Standards Compliance report.

Plan of action
A plan detailing the action(s) that an organization will take in order to come into compliance with a JCAHO standard. A plan of action must be completed at the element of performance (EP) level, and for each EP a measure of success (MOS) must be completed.

Priority focus areas (PFAs)
Processes, systems, or structures in a health care organization that can significantly impact the provision of safe, high-quality care. The PFAs are as follows:

- Assessment and Care/Services
- Communication
- Credentialed Practitioners
- Equipment Use
- Infection Control

- Information Management
- Medication Management
- Organizational Structure
- Orientation and Training
- Rights and Ethics
- Physical Environment
- Quality Improvement Expertise and Activity
- Patient Safety
- Staffing
- Analytical Procedures (replaces Assessment and Care/Services in laboratories)

Priority Focus Process (PFP)
The process for standardizing the priorities for sampling during an organization's survey based on information collected about the organization prior to survey. The process also helps to focus the survey on areas that are critical to that organization's patient safety and quality-of-care processes. Examples of such information may include, but are not limited to, data from the organization's e-App; data from JCAHO's Quality Monitoring System, including complaints; data collected from external sources, such as MedPAR (Medicare Provider Analysis and Review) data; performance measurement data; and previous survey results.

Priority Focus Tool (PFT)
An automated tool that supports the Priority Focus Process through the use of algorithms, or sets of rules, to transform a health care organization's data into information that guides the survey process.

Recommendation
A survey finding cited in an organization's Accreditation Report that needs to be addressed in the organization's Evidence of Standards Compliance report.

Requirement for improvement
A survey finding cited in an organization's Accreditation Report that needs to be addressed in the organization's Evidence of Standards Compliance (ESC) report. Failure to address a requirement for improvement after two opportunities will result in a recommendation to place the organization in Conditional Accreditation.

Shared Visions–New Pathways
A JCAHO initiative to progressively sharpen the focus of the accreditation process on care systems critical to the safety and quality of patient, client, or resident care.

Standard
A statement that defines the performance expectations, structures, or processes that must be in place for an organization to provide safe and high-quality care, treatment, and services.

Standards Interpretation Group
The function of the Standards Interpretation Group is to identify, develop, maintain, and communicate the meaning of all Joint Commission standards to all customers—such as accredited organizations—surveyors, Central Office staff, and other interested parties.

Supplemental finding
A finding that triggers a partial score at the Element of Performance (EP) level, but within a standard that is still identified as compliant and that is not required to be addressed in an organization's Evidence of Standards Compliance (ESC) but should be addressed by the organization internally. A supplemental finding will also be factored into an organization's Priority Focus Process at its next survey.

System tracer
An activity during the on-site survey devoted to evaluating high-priority safety and quality-of-care issues on a systemwide basis throughout the organization. Examples of such issues include infection control, medication management, and use of data.

Tracer methodology
A process surveyors use during the on-site survey to analyze an organization's systems, with particular attention to identified priority focus areas, by following individual patients, clients, or residents through the organization's health care process as experienced by the patients, residents, or clients. Depending on the health care setting, this process may require surveyors to visit multiple care units, departments or areas within an organization, or a single care unit to "trace" the care rendered to the patient, resident, or client.

INDEX

B

C

D

E

L

M

N

O

S

T